Duck Summer

MY ODYSSEY AS A DIALYSIS PATIENT

Derrick,

Thank you for your support. I look forward to any comments. Hope things are going well for you.

Angelene Ladd
1/23/16

Printed by CreateSpace

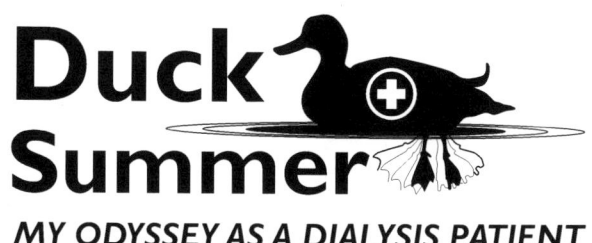

MY ODYSSEY AS A DIALYSIS PATIENT

Angelene J. Hall
www.angelenejhall.com
www.ducksummer.com

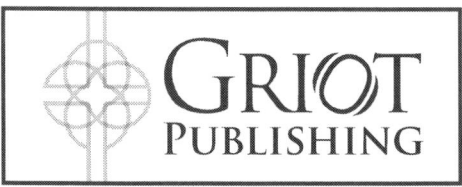

Cincinnati, Ohio
2014
www.griotpublishing.com

DUCK SUMMER: *MY ODYSSEY AS A DIALYSIS PATIENT*

Copyright © November 2014, Angelene J. Hall

Cover art by Griot Marketing Services, LLC
Copyright November 2014 Cincinnati, OH

All rights reserved. Published in United States
by
Griot Publishing, LLC.

No part of this document or the related files may be reproduced or transmitted in any form, by any means (electronic, photocopying, recording, or otherwise) without the prior written permission of the publisher.

ISBN 978-0-9862576-0-5

Dedication and Acknowledgements

To God, my compass and my strength, thank You for allowing me to travel this journey and live to tell the story.

To the spirits of my mother and father, I know you must be aware of how much your presence has meant to me as I worked on DUCK SUMMER. Thank you.

Leslie, your support and encouragement provided much of the impetus for me to continue to work on the manuscript when the enthusiasm waned. Thank you for always being there to remind me of my goal.

Binta, thank you for reading my manuscript, providing your invaluable commentary, and insisting that I have a story worth telling. Your support is affirmation of the stories in print and those still smoldering in my thoughts.

B.J., thank you for your steadfast encouragement, support and eagerness always to read and comment on my writing.

Katherine, for years, you have read my writing with a critical eye. I appreciate your consistency, dedication, and commitment.

Ann and Roger, remember all the days, weeks, and eventually years we sat in our workshops critiquing each other's work and insisting on the refinement of our writing? Thank you. I especially you for your agreeing to hold the workshops at my home after I began dialysis.

To all of my healthcare providers—physicians, nurses, social workers, and dialysis staff, thank you. I would like to give a special thanks to my primary care physician, nephrologists, vascular surgeons, endocrinologists and transplant surgeons.

Finally, to all those currently on dialysis, you are never far from my thoughts. I pray for your wellness.

Content

Dedication and Acknowledgements

Prologue

Chapter 1 • JUST A REGULAR APPOINTMENT	1
Chapter 2 • A CLEAN HEART, O GOD	8
Chapter 3 • OMINOUS NEWS	25
Chapter 4 • IN SEARCH OF GOD	34
Chapter 5 • SEAGULLS AND ITALIAN ICE	45
Chapter 6 • THE HOSPITAL MAZE	52
Chapter 7 • A NUCLEAR EXPLOSION	66
Chapter 8 • A JOURNEY OF ONE'S OWN	72
Chapter 9 • FISTULAS, CATHETERS, AND GRAFTS	85
Chapter 10 • WATER, WATER, EVERYWHERE	99
Chapter 11 • AGH! DIALYSIS AND HAIR LOSS, TOO	104
Chapter 12 • A GLIMPSE OF DIALYSIS CULTURE	118
Chapter 13 • THE KIDNEY FACTORY: DIALYSIS FOR PROFIT AND THE OUTPATIENT CLINICS	128
Chapter 14 • KIDNEY TRANSPLANTS	138
Epilogue	142
The Author	144

Prologue

I could almost see the end of the tortuous trail. Images of parked bikes, motor scooters, and people roaming around the Popsicle stands shimmered through the blazing heat. Hazy impressions of dancing children faded in and out of my view, and my friend, whom I could always outrun, leaped ahead as if she had wings. Although I wasn't sure what was happening to me, I knew it wasn't good. For years, I had taken pride in my long distance running, and now I was struggling behind someone who rarely walked, and certainly had no running experience.

Though the tenacious forces fought feverishly against me, I was determined to get to the end of the trail. But with each labored stride, my legs became increasingly heavier, my breathing labored, and the faint ringing in my ears was alarming. I should have stopped, but I refused to surrender to the horrendous demands of this unusual fatigue. I trudged on. By the time I reached the car, my throat was as dry as dust, my tongue clung to the roof of my mouth, and I panted like a woman in labor.

I didn't run again that summer. I didn't have the energy. Now I know that all along I was really quite ill, and it has taken almost a decade for me to put the things that happened that summer of 1998 in some kind of perspective. This is it. This is the story of my "Duck Summer," which lingered for six years as I underwent kidney dialysis.

Chapter 1

JUST A REGULAR APPOINTMENT

It was 1998. May. I had my regular appointment with my primary care physician, whom I had been seeing for over two decades.

Unlike some patients who remain with a doctor until either the doctor or the patient dies, or the doctor ceases practicing medicine and begins to sell pharmaceuticals, I don't think I ever had the same kind of blind loyalty when it comes to my health. Although switching doctors is not as simple as switching hair stylists, unsatisfactory doctors don't deserve any more allegiance than unsatisfactory hair stylists. If the doctor practices bad medicine—writing prescriptions that have nothing to do with the illness, running patients through the office like an assembly line, ordering unnecessary tests, and demonstrating poor people skills, then he or she is not for me.

However, I had remained with this doctor because she was very good and proved to be one of my greatest blessings. A brilliant internist with a messianic bedside manner, she was a guardian angel, not just to me, but to her many other patients as well. With her extremely cautious nature, she has saved me from several potential health crises because of her keen observance and her rigorous follow-through. Always staying abreast of medical problems, she remembers all medications, coordinates her patients' medical care, responds expeditiously to phone calls, and treats her patients as people, instead of a particular illness or chart number.

As an internist, she recommends the specialists and makes sure her patients are able to get a timely appointment with the suggested physician. Problems with insurance companies aside, she works effectively with the system to ensure her patients receive the best medical help. This kind of dedicated proficiency is especially important since medicine is assaulted by exorbitant costs, choking controls by insurance companies, draconian demands on physicians for increasing productivity (more patients in less time), and many other bureaucratic barriers to good healthcare.

My appointment was scheduled for 11:00 AM. Usually, there is at least a twenty-minute wait because this doctor is thorough and uses more time with each patient than the office manager schedules or recommends. This time, however, the office was empty and in less than five minutes, the nurse called me to the scales. I always hated these check-up appointments because the older I get, the more I realize the potential for health problems.

In my younger days, I rarely went to a doctor because I assumed they were for the sick. Even after I learned I might have an ailment that couldn't be treated with castor oil or dogwood tea, I put trust in the vitality of youth. However, as the increasing years began to manifest themselves in a gravitational pull on my body that sent a shock through my system, I found myself in the doctor's office more frequently than I ever imagined.

Thus, with fear and trembling, I approached the scales, stripping of all non-essentials--shoes, earrings, watch, belt, eyeglasses and any other accessories that might carry unnecessary weight. After getting the weight out of the way, I saw the nurse come towards me again, this time with a needle, and I broke out in another sweat. With extremely small veins, I had run into too many nurses who apparently received their training at an auto mechanic school, and I always dreaded the experience. Because blood tests were the most critical part of the check-up, these nightmarish encounters caused the greatest anxiety, as they determined whether I was in for grief or elation.

*****

DUCK SUMMER: *MY ODYSSEY AS A DIALYSIS PATIENT*

My first acquaintance with the needle as it related to my kidneys had come twenty-five years earlier when I was diagnosed with a renal disease—chronic membraneous proliferative glomerulonephritis. I thought I had the flu since I experienced headaches, fever, nausea, and an aggravating backache. When aspirin and a few home remedies didn't work and I felt progressively worse, I went to the emergency room where I was eventually admitted to the hospital. When urine tests found microscopic traces of protein and blood, the physician recommended I see a urologist. Subsequent blood tests and eventually a kidney biopsy indicated a slightly elevated creatinine level and a scarred kidney.

For years, I visited nephrologists who initially checked blood and protein levels in my urine, and later evaluated my kidney function through blood tests. It took a day, sometimes two, to get the results, and I always worried about the kidney function levels.

I loathed the waiting. Between the times the nurses drilled into my arm, finally drawing blood, and the doctor got in touch with me, the anxiety was maddening. For more than twenty years, I had no symptoms discernable to me. Very careful with my health, I paid particular attention to diet and exercise. Vegetables became the focus of my diet, and I spent considerable time exercising—running, walking, aerobic dancing, and some weight training.

My physicians and I credited the longevity of my kidney function to the grace of God, diet, exercise, and a simple lifestyle. Actually, with more than twenty years after the initial diagnosis and no severe consequences, I had begun to think complete renal failure might not be in my future. I had even started to feel less angst about my doctor's visits until I developed high blood pressure, a known cause and effect of kidney disease.

High blood pressure stemming from the renal complications was a clear indication that my kidneys were on the decline. I was back on the seesaw—anxious about test results one week, struggling with despair the next. Would my blood pressure be normal or borderline high? What about the sodium level? Triglycerides? Potassium? Would the BUN (blood urea nitrogen) indicate an even bigger problem? Would the creatinine show an elevation since the last test? A normal level for an adult over forty is somewhere between a .9 and 1.2, and mine had already reached 4.8 a few years before complete failure. Frequent blood tests had indicated a gradual increase of the creatinine level over the last five or six years, but I was still living a relatively normal life, despite the occasional bouts with an elevated blood pressure and an abnormal creatinine level.

Kidney failure is scary. When I learned that ESRD (End Stage Renal Disease) affected almost every aspect of the body, I lived with a healthy dose of paranoia. Blood pressure, lung and heart strength, nerves, body chemistries, digestion, emotions, bones, appetite, and other equally important health matters dominated my thoughts. I checked my blood pressure daily, monitored my appetite, and worried whenever my ankles or fingers appeared swollen. At visits with the physician, I compared current kidney panels to the most recent, questioned chemistries I didn't understand, and tried unsuccessfully to figure out how long it would be before I would have to confront *the machine*.

I was slowly and silently becoming a nervous wreck.

I remember some of the horror stories I heard from people already on dialysis, once I realized it was imminent. A church member, already a dialysis patient, said I would be okay the day after dialysis, but on treatment day, I would probably feel as if I had been hit by a freighter and might even be unable to function. Another told me he exercised during the first few weeks of treatments, but shortly thereafter became too exhausted to continue. Too frequently I even heard stories about incompetence, sexual dysfunction, heart disease, debilitating fatigue, breathing difficulties and other life-altering problems.

DUCK SUMMER: *MY ODYSSEY AS A DIALYSIS PATIENT*

*****

In the early afternoon of May 18, 1998, the nurse drew the blood, took my pressure and put my file in the rack on the back of the examining room door. "The doctor will be with you in a moment," she said, pushing the door almost closed.

Sitting in the tiny windowless room where the smell of disinfectant burned the inside of my nose, I could hear sounds from the outside waiting room as clear as if we were all together. The nurses' shoes swishing over the carpet, the *brri, brri, brri* of the phone, the receptionist's high-pitched voice bouncing against the wall, and somebody's distant snoring, all settled into the pit of my stomach. How many times during the course of a day, I wondered, do I sit and wait for something that will inevitably affect the course of my life? How many minutes ticked slowly by while I thumbed through magazines focusing on celebrities and their weight loss? What about the pee-colored patterns on the boring green wallpaper? I always hated those "medicinal" colors and often imagined more colorful lifelike designs, something like robins and blue jays hovering around petunias under an afternoon sun.

This cloudy afternoon, I added a cardinal to the wallpaper and planted some red salvia, both which completely chased away any remaining gloom and gave the paper an even greater vibrancy. Finally, satisfied with my imaginary surroundings, I clasped my hands under my chin and began a silent prayer that the tests would show improvement or at the very least, no changes.

My doctor entered the room. Always able to compensate for the long wait with her calming voice, her reassuring hands, and, ironically, her enduring patience, she made me feel guilty for my impatience and restlessness. Moreover, I knew she had been with other patients who were equally apprehensive and I chastised myself for selfishness and insensitivity.

During the check-up, she answered my questions promptly and with no sign of annoyance that I had asked the same questions at the last several visits. "Is it possible that my creatinine might stabilize? What has been the percentage of change in the BUN over the last six months? Do I really need to be concerned about complete kidney failure? What if I drank only a half can of diet cola a day?"

Examining my lower back, under my arms, and checking my reflexes, she spoke calmly. "Well, you know . . . if it were left up to me, you would have already been on dialysis." She reached for her chart and began flipping through the pages. "With these numbers . . ." She shook her head as she perused the test results. "I don't know, but I don't think it will be long."

She placed the chart on the small desk. "So how do you feel today?" She began pressing my neck with her fingers.

"I feel okay." I tilted my head back for her to examine my throat.

She continued to press on my neck while we asked about each other's family. "Would you stand up for me, please?" The conversation lulled me as she continued to explore. Massaging the front of my neck with her thumbs, she took a step back from me and looked with questioning eyes. "Is your neck swollen?" She felt it again.

"No," I said, adamantly. I am very aware of any changes in my body and I was certain there was no unusual swelling. I felt a hot flash coming on and since I was nude from the waist up, I would have given almost anything to snatch a tissue from the box to soak the perspiration from under my breasts.

"Are you having any trouble swallowing?" She was still probing.

"No." I dropped my head and breathed, trying to cool my burning chest, which by now, was dripping with moisture. "Is there a problem?" I took another deep breath, already beginning to feel sorry

I had asked the question. As much as I loved her, I grew annoyed by her constant probing. Why couldn't she just leave this alone? There was nothing wrong with my throat.

She surveyed my neck again. "You sure you haven't noticed any swelling?"

"Yes ... I mean, no, I haven't noticed." I felt my throat. Nothing.

"Is there any soreness?"

"No."

She sat down and began to write on the chart. "I feel a thickness there, and just to be on the safe side, I'm going to write this order for you to go to the hospital to get an ultrasound."

"When?"

"As soon as possible." She smiled and handed me the prescription. "Now, don't start worrying. Most of the time, these kinds of things are nothing, really. We just have to check them out. Better to be safe," she said in a singsong tone.

I left the office thinking, God, why do I have to do this? Not another test. My doctor was certainly living up to her reputation. Any suspicion of an abnormality, no matter how minor, is cause for further examination. Since 1984, I had probably undergone every conceivable test at least twice. My doctor had recommended CT scans, bone scans, colonoscopies, upper GI's, endoscopies, MRI's and all kinds of blood tests. In spite of her predisposition to frequent patient testing, both patients and doctors have praised her for the meticulous care she provides. Moreover, her attention to physical detail had ultimately contributed to saving lives. With this information in mind, I tried not to complain as I headed to another one of those dreaded labs.

Chapter 2

A CLEAN HEART, O GOD

The world was tightening its grip on my spirit. I had made a commitment to serve as keynote speaker for a community council banquet scheduled three weeks after my appointment with the doctor. Moving through the revolving doors at the medical center, I felt as if I were plummeting into quicksand. The council wanted a speech, the doctor wanted an ultrasound, the University wanted final exam grades, and the students wanted A's for D work. Everybody wanted something from me, leaving me with no time or energy to figure out what I wanted for myself.

I may not have known what I wanted, but I certainly knew what I needed and didn't need. It seems so simple now, but then my exams, the grades, and particularly the presentation were monkeys on my back—each one trying to out-scratch the other. What I didn't need was the gorilla, another medical test to worry about. But no matter how much I griped, I always followed up on the doctor's recommendations, and this time would be no different. I scheduled the ultrasound for Thursday, three days after the visit with the doctor.

I was familiar with the technician who performed these tests, as I had been to this section of the hospital many times. The tall freckled-faced redhead with lipstick matching her hair was pleasant enough to allay my fears, but apparently not at liberty to give me any details about my throat. "Does it look okay?" I mumbled.

"What?" She ran the scope over my neck.

"My throat," I said when she took a break to re-gel the instrument.

She smiled. "Your doctor will give you all the results."

Her tone was formal, and I knew no more than I did at first.

I never understood why technicians couldn't divulge the slightest bit of information, especially since the patient had the right to know. I reasoned that if this white-coated woman read the film inaccurately, then she could have been held responsible for misinforming the patient. But, if she did understand, she might have been prohibited from exposing the results, since she was not the physician. The situation was exasperating.

What often added to my frustration was the length of time it took the radiologists to read the test, get the information to the doctor, and ultimately to me. Why was the patient the last to know? And why did it take so long to get the results?

After the ultrasound of my throat, I had to put the declining function of my kidneys on the back burner for a while. So much was happening and I had so many responsibilities, I felt like flinging it all into the Ohio River and pretending I was someone else.

Though I wished temporarily to turn my back on my problems, I knew I would never be able to do so. Chucking life, even in desperate times, was simply not me. Thus, I prepared the final exams for my classes, figured out how I would get them graded, and then began to reflect on the speech. The only reason I even considered making a presentation was that the request had come from a man who had been my student at the University during my first few years as a professor.

I selected my topic carefully while trying to stay within the guidelines set by the organization. "A Clean Heart, A Right Spirit: The Community, Leaders, and The New Millennium" sounded massive, but I figured I could work with it.

I mulled over the speech because I wanted it to touch those in the audience at a deeper level than most community talks, although I also wondered how a 15 or 20 minute presentation would make much difference to anybody. Half of these people would not pay attention and the other half would not remember a thing I said. How could I make this gathering more than just a group of us coming together for a couple of hours, chatting superficially, chomping through a cliché-chicken dinner, and patting each other on the back?

I wanted my presentation to shake people up and make them think about their ability to contribute to a world that I sometimes thought was on its way to hell. I craved something that would transform Cincinnati's Black social circles into unswerving activists. As I think back on it now, I must have subconsciously transferred my anxiety over my health into a need to reach out to people.

In the weeks I had been meandering through the medical maze, I had begun to watch others and myself from a growing distance. Constantly accompanied by fear and aloneness, I had the nagging urge to talk about people wrestling with anxiety, isolation, and the scariness of uncertainty. I also wanted to talk about how to address the panic accompanying the realization of how little control we have in life, how one day we might have plans firmly in place and the next, we are forced to reorder our priorities.

I think I was searching for affirmation that people did, indeed, give a damn about others and their struggles. Would the social workers, the councilpersons, the ministers, and teachers go into the new millennium with a determination to make a recognizable difference in our neighborhoods? Would I even care, especially now that I stood at the cliff of sanity, struggling not to fall?

I forced the ultrasound to the back of my mind and concentrated on the speech for several days. Reviewing the language, and checking to see if my points were clear, I made sure I'd used my chosen scripture effectively. "Give me a clean heart, O God, and put a new and right spirit within me." Psalm 51, Verse 10 echoed in my head like a spiritual as I prepared my presentation, challenging those who have accepted positions of responsibility in the community to recognize our potential to make changes.

*****

On Saturday morning, eleven days before the banquet, as I was making some final revisions, the nurse called to tell me my family physician wanted me to see an ENT (Ear, Nose, and Throat) specialist.

"Oh Lord," I mumbled over the phone. My body grew hot, heating from the inside. "What is it now?"

It had been almost two weeks since the ultrasound and I had struggled to put the test out of my mind. "Did the test show something?"

"Yes," she said, obviously trying to lessen the impact of the news. "There is some kind of growth in your neck."

"What kind of growth? Where in my neck?" My hands began to sweat and I noticed perspiration on the keyboard. Instinctively, I walked my fingers over my throat. "Can it be something bad?"

"Now take it easy," she said reassuringly. "It's around the throat area. Most of the time these things are nothing but cysts. However, we will want to check it out just to be on the safe side. It's just a precaution, nothing but a precaution."

"Well, does that mean . . .?"

"Aw, don't worry. If there's a problem, this is early and we can take care of it."

"What d'you mean, a problem? What kind of problem could it be?"

"It's probably just a cyst, and that can be removed with ease."

I couldn't think fast enough to ask any more questions. Moreover, I knew she couldn't answer what I really wanted to know—whether or not I had a serious problem.

As soon as I hung up the phone, I ran to the bathroom and spent much of the rest of the morning looking at my throat. Pressing it on each side in an effort to feel some ill-defined growth, I opened my mouth wide to see if I could notice anything different. I couldn't believe that on top of my apprehension about the upcoming banquet, and my concern that one day I might not be able to pee, I had something else to worry about.

While I never really got the test out of my mind, I told myself it wouldn't show anything problematic, and I didn't even bother to call the doctor about the results. Yet, there *was* a problem, and now I had to wait until the following week before I could see the specialist.

When I did see him, I learned that there was indeed a growth, and it was defined as having a "malignant potential."

"If the report says, 'malignant potential'," I asked, "does that mean it could be can ... cancer?"

The doctor, an Asian who seemed to be a patient man, immediately recognized my anxiety. "Cancer?" He raised his glasses and looked at the report. "Not necessarily. We just have to remove it to be on the side of caution." He gave my hand an encouraging pat. "It's going to be all right. My secretary will schedule the procedure before you leave."

His hand was warm and undemanding, but it didn't make me feel any better. When he walked out of the room, I wanted to reach out and grab his arm the way a child hangs onto a parent when she senses danger. I didn't want him to leave me with no answers and another waiting period. Unsure of what questions to ask, I wanted him to wait until I had time to figure them out.

The clerk scheduled the surgery exactly one week from that day. Before pre-admission testing, I had my interview with the Registrar, a fortyish anorexic-looking woman, who seemed to care only about whether or not I had insurance. "Where do you work? Do you have insurance? Is it in your name or your husband's? Do you have your insurance card with you? May I see it? Is this the most recent?"

The questions rolled off the registrar's tongue like a pre-recorded message. Add that to her expressionless face and she looked like a robotic mannequin.

"What would have happened if I had come in bleeding profusely . . . my arm hanging from my shoulder by one bloody tendon?"

"We'd still have to get that card." She blew a couple of yellowish brown strands of hair from her plastic face, but she never looked up from the computer, and I was still as invisible to her as the gnat whizzing about her coffee cup.

"Do you have any advanced directives?"

"No."

"Here," she said handing me some forms on blue paper. "Read this when you get a chance." She then pointed to another form. "Sign here, then go to pre-admission testing."

The pre-admission testing included a blood pressure reading, blood and urine tests, weight and height measurement, an EKG, and a general physical. When I tiptoed into the room for the EKG and physical, I bumped into the physician, another Asian, this one a woman. Already anxious and plagued by a sense of dread, the last thing I needed was a physician who probably had about as much in common with me as my sister did to the Queen of England. The other problem, of course, was whether or not she spoke clear English.

A woman of forty or fifty-something (it was hard to tell), she appeared quite nonchalant as she went about examining my reflexes, my chest and back, and then hooking me up to the EKG machine.

Since her English pronunciation was much better than some Americans I know, I relaxed somewhat. Maybe she would say something that would calm my fears about the upcoming procedure. But I didn't even know if she knew why I was there. She simply followed the routine—questioning me about smoking, drinking, previous hospitalizations, and my list of medications.

Asians, I thought. What do they know, especially about African Americans? Why should I expect her to reassure me? I am just another patient in this stupid faded gown and I am nobody special to this woman. What does she care? And why should she? She's probably picked up all the myths about us that permeate this country. Huh, I thought, we have some stories about her kind, too—come over here, get welfare and the next thing you know they are doctors.

In spite of myself, I chuckled. Here I was, confronting these major health challenges and yet, thinking about what the two of us might think of each other. How stupid. She might not be thinking of me at all. However, as much as I tried to squash any xenophobic thoughts, I visualized American medical professionals leaving domestic patients to the Asians in favor of a spot on T.V.

By the time my tests were finished, I had worked myself into an emotional frazzle. I imagined jumping from the table, grabbing the doctor's soft pink neck, and shaking her. "See *me!* See *me!*" I wanted to scream. In the vision, my eyes bulged as I yelled through my teeth. Beginning to pee on herself, the doctor jerked away from me and ran screaming down the hall.

"We're finished, Mrs. Hall," the doctor said with an abruptness that snapped me back to reality.

"Do you pray?" These words tumbled wildly from my mouth.

"Yes, I do." She smiled from one side of her mouth with no sign of surprise at my question.

"Will you pray for me?" My desperation had taken control of my behavior and I was like a woman falling off a cliff, grabbing for anyone or anything.

"Yes, Mrs. Hall," she said and reached for my hand. "Yes, I will."

I sat on the table for a few minutes, my mouth parted in shame, staring at this woman and wondering if she could sense my embarrassment and fear. For a minute, I wanted her to lead me to some far away exotic place where there would be no hospitals, no pre-admissions testing, and no waiting for anything. "Thank you," I said. "Thank you very much."

The time between pre-admission testing and the surgery passed quickly and the next thing I knew I was awake and talking to the surgeon.

"Everything went fine," he said. "Nothing to worry about."

"Was it cancerous?" I hated the sound of the question. It reminded me of relatives I had lost from the disease. *Cancer* had always been a scary word.

"We won't know that until we get the report back from the pathologist. We also removed part of the thyroid."

"Why?" My throat felt as if it had swollen closed over thumbtacks.

"To test it." He fingered the I-V tubing.

I tried to swallow, but the pain wouldn't allow it.

"When you removed the tissue," I muttered, saliva filling my mouth. When I tried to spit, it spilled from the side of my mouth and the doctor pressed a couple of tissues against it.

"You need to rest," he said. "The anesthesia hasn't even worn off yet. I'll be back later this afternoon." He started towards the door.

"Can-cer?" I strained to get the word out. "I mean, did it look like those you have seen before?" I breathed in spurts and fell back against the pillow. "That . . . that were cancerous?" I was trying to frame the question to get something close to a definitive response.

I knew my surgeon had been in the business long enough to recognize cancer when he saw it. I'd researched him when I learned he would be the one performing the procedure, so I knew more about him than he would ever know about me. He was one of the top throat surgeons in the business, but he refused to hazard a guess. Damn, I thought. Doctors! They don't want to speculate about a damn thing, and in the meantime, the patient wrestles with all this doubt and uncertainty.

He returned to the bed and tapped me on my hand. His hands were just as warm and undemanding as they were that day in his office. "Don't worry. We'll know everything in a few days." He spoke as if he knew what I had been thinking. "In the meantime, I'm going to write this prescription for your throat, and you can go home tomorrow. See me in my office one week from today."

I don't remember how long I slept before I awakened in a double room in the hospital where another woman lay in the bed adjacent to mine. Lying on my back staring at the ceiling, I listened to her conversation with her daughters.

"Yeah, I'm so glad this wasn't nothing but a cyst." I heard the bed squeaking as she apparently turned.

"We are too, Mama. We prayed."

"Yes, Jesus. Thank you. Thank you, Jesus."

"And Mama, he already removed the cyst?" Another woman raised the question.

I turned my body to face the side of the room of the woman

and her family.

"Yes, baby. They already removed the cyst and I'm fine. Just a little sore throat. To tell you the truth, I'm hungry."

I closed my eyes and soon heard the voice of my surgeon. He was talking with the woman, reassuring her she could eat anything she wanted and go home the next morning as soon as he could get her dismissed. "No cancer," he said. "You're doing fine, and I'll see you first thing in the morning."

In order not to have to talk, even if the woman or her daughters did want to be friendly, I pretended I was asleep. I actually fell asleep and awakened to the smell of a burger and fries. Still lying in the same position, I squinted enough to see what was going on, and noticed the woman sitting up in bed, her large frame propped with pillows. A tray with fries, a huge burger, a large drink, and a fruit pie rested on her lap. The woman, only hours from surgery, was chowing down on fast food.

I turned on my back and stared at the cell-like indentations in the ceiling panels. Listening to the crunch crunch of the woman's chewing the fries and later the long slurp from the cola, I feigned waking up, stretched and looked over at the celebration.

"Hi," I said.

"Hey there," the woman responded, manipulating food from her jaw and swallowing.

"I see we're roommates." I didn't know what else to say.

"Yeah." Trying to squelch a belch, she blew gas from her puckered lips. "I just had surgery early this morning."

"Me too. I'm glad it's over." I wanted to know why she received her reports so quickly and I still didn't have mine. I couldn't let her know, however, that I had heard her talking when I pretended to be asleep. "Sure takes a long time to hear anything."

"Not for me, honey. The doctor just came in earlier and told me everything was fine. I had a cyst, right here." The woman pointed to her throat and picked up a fry.

I started to worry about why I wouldn't get my reports for a while. Maybe the nodule was in a different location. Maybe it was a different kind. I couldn't bear watching the woman picnicking in the hospital room another minute, so I closed my eyes.

Although I was still groggy from the pre and post-operative medicines, I knew exactly the source of my developing anger. I was about to come to the conclusion that justice must be as sparse as adolescents with good manners. My roommate had just enjoyed one of fast food's epicurean delights and seemingly ignored the potential of adding two or three pounds to the possibly two hundred and fifty she was already carrying. She had come into the hospital, gotten the result of her biopsy, which was benign, and had been given the permission to go home.

I, on the other hand, had learned nothing of my biopsy, was barely able to talk, much less eat, and had to wait almost a week before I would learn my fate. I would never have eaten a hamburger and fries, nor drank a big cola for any reason. The saturated fat, trans fat, sugar, salt and calories were poison to me, and I had to watch my weight like a model. Running five miles every morning, I thought I had an insurance policy against illness. Yet, compared to the woman in the next bed, who obviously had a less fastidious approach to life, I was the one struggling from the procedure. I tried not to think about the kidney problem because I couldn't handle but one threat at a time.

Three days later, I had an early morning appointment with my family physician. I was her first patient. It had occurred to me to cancel because the most important date was the one with the specialist. However, I thought perhaps I should go ahead and see her because she had the kind of reassuring manner I needed, especially now. I waited for her about twenty minutes in a room that was unusually cold. Wrapping my arms around myself, I sat bent until I heard the click of the door.

When the doctor entered the examination room, she gave me a hug, which is often her custom.

"Hi!" She sat on her stool and scooted closer to me. "I got the report back from the surgeon," she spoke slowly, thumbing through the folder. Her voice was somber. A few seconds passed where the only sound was her flipping the pages of the chart.

I tensed. "Is everything okay?"

She raised her eyes from the chart and shook her head.

"Is it can . . .?" I still couldn't get the word out.

"Yes," she said as if she were talking to a child who had gotten lost from its mother. She took my hands and looked into my eyes.

I gasped. It seemed I couldn't breathe. I knew I must have heard her wrong. "It . . . it . . . is it . . .it . . . cancer?" I repeated.

She nodded and squeezed my hand.

"Oh God! Oh God!" Snatching my hand away from her, I jumped from the chair. "Oh God! Oh God! Not that! No!" I began to sway from side to side, as if the movements would rewind the clock and none of this would be happening.

"Thyroid cancer can be taken care of," she said, reaching and trying to still me in front of her. "If you've got to have a cancer, it's the least invasive, especially the kind you have."

"But cancer, oh God!" I took a deep breath. "Am I going to die?" I began to cry. "Cancer is dea . . . It's . . . Is that . . .?

"No! Shh!" She tried to assure me. "No! No! I want you to see the specialist. I talked to him and he gave me the results, but I told him

I wanted to tell you myself. I stopped by his office before I came in to get the results."

I could not even thank my doctor for her concern. I was devastated. I had cancer--the thing I had most feared, the thing we all fear. It was the thing people whispered about when I was growing up, the thing the old people referred to as "C" because they couldn't bring themselves to say the word. I was dazed; none of this was happening. It could not be happening. I couldn't have this dreaded thing, this thing that changes strong healthy people into crumbling fetal-shaped weaklings with no hair.

What in the hell is thyroid cancer? Thyroid? What does a thyroid do, anyway? As I sat in her office, her soft comforting voice floating past me like harp music, I wondered why, of all the people in the world, was this happening to me? What had I done? For years, I had tried to live a healthy life. I had quit smoking more than fifteen years ago. I ate right. I exercised. I prayed. I checked on the old people. I worked in church. What else could I do? I didn't deserve thyroid cancer.

And what about my kidney function? Did the kidneys cause the thyroid problem? Did the thyroid affect the kidneys?

It was that Friday in my doctor's office that I started on a journey that led me through a desert of my faith. That day marked the beginning of a long spiritual dry spell, a period where I struggled to maintain my relationship with God. Would a relationship with Him mean He would shield me from some of the problems we face or just help me to cope with them?

I knew there were numerous people who had a strong connection with God, yet had certainly borne their share of crosses. I had been raised to accept the mystery of God without question, but with my recent health issues, I was beset by uncertainties. Where was He? Did He hear me when I prayed? Of all the people in the world, was

I worth His taking time to listen to me? Given that I couldn't respond satisfactorily to my own queries, I felt I was losing my spiritual grounding.

Fearful that God would see me as a fair-weather Christian, I wanted to be at peace with Him. I wanted to be one of His chosen, one whom He would look upon with favor. Imagining an angry God was not an option, especially given the dilemmas I was currently facing. Yet, I couldn't help but wonder if I were *selected* for thyroid cancer and kidney failure, or did these things just happen arbitrarily.

Weighted by the information and the burdensome questions, I left the doctor's office feeling as if I were climbing a steep mountain in lead boots. The joints in my legs rebelled against each step which seemed to cement itself to the sidewalk. Tired and disoriented, I finally reached the car, exhausted and out of breath. For a moment, I felt as if I were watching a video of my body propped against the car, gasping for breath.

When a car horn blew, I came out of my trance, still breathing heavily, beads of perspiration streaming down the sides of my face and dripping from my nose. "Thyroid cancer," I uttered repeatedly, as I got into the car. Inside, the heat was thick enough to chew and I snatched a handkerchief from my purse, looked into the rearview mirror and wiped my face. That afternoon, in the smoldering heat of my car, I leaned my head against the steering wheel and cried.

I couldn't remember a time I'd felt more alone. My mother was in a different state. My husband and daughter were both at work, and my closest friends were either out of town, inaccessible by phone, or at that time of the afternoon, in class. For a while, I sat in the car with the windows cracked just enough to prevent suffocation. I dried my eyes and took a deep breath. I had to pull myself together because this was *my* news, nobody else's, and the world would still go on. The sun would still rise in the east the next day and it would set in the west.

I backed the car out of the parking lot of the medical building. Out on the sidewalk, some students, apparently from one of the neighboring sorority houses, passed by with earphones plastered to their ears. One of them stopped to do a jig to the silent music and the other threw her head back in laughter. They were happy. And why wouldn't they be? They didn't have cancer; they weren't worried about their kidneys. Stopping at the end of the driveway, I tilted my head towards the sky. God had painted dull bluish gray clouds above, a haze that shut out the sun, and had breathed humidity that hung over the earth like a tenacious fog.

*****

The day I learned I had thyroid cancer was also the day I was scheduled to speak at the banquet. Only three days after surgery on the left side of my thyroid, my throat was swollen and raw, and I sounded as if I had a mouth full of marbles. I probably should have reneged, but I had put too much work into the speech not to present it. Hence, the only thing to do was get dressed, swallow a couple of pain pills, and head to the hotel.

The event had drawn the usual crowd from the business, social service, education and religious communities. Leaders from community councils, the Urban League, and various churches meandered through the oval room, chatting and sipping drinks. Several people from various agencies, the city council, and one or two self-help representatives wandered along the table of hors d'oeuvres, occasionally maneuvering their plate to one hand in order to embrace one of the banquet leaders with the other.

A young high school girl with dark lipstick and a black glistening Marge Simpson hairdo met my husband and me at the door and led us to our seats. As I followed her, my stomach reeled and I feared I might throw up. I held my breath, wishing I could simply swallow my engorged tonsils.

DUCK SUMMER: *MY ODYSSEY AS A DIALYSIS PATIENT*

After sitting at the front for several minutes and shaking a few hands, I got up and roamed the room, swallowing with difficulty when my mouth filled with water, and smiling when anyone approached me. All the time I prayed no one would stop to engage me in any conversation requiring more than a pleasant nod. Planning for the drool threatening to expose itself if I dared utter a word, I snatched a tissue from my purse and lightly covered my mouth.

I was miserable and found no relief in people-watching, something I usually enjoy. Even women in glimmering dresses that shimmered against audacious hips and thighs, promenading around the banquet room, pretending to search for their tables, provided no humor. The upscale-suited men, chins pointed towards the chandeliers, and hands pompously grasping their lapels, didn't even get a cynical nod, not to mention a scathing thought.

Looking over the crowd through watering eyes, I wondered what these people would think if they knew I had just had a biopsy for thyroid cancer and could barely talk. My throat hurt when I breathed, and with my ballooned tonsils, there was no way I could eat. When dinner came, I pushed the food around my plate and pretended. The tea I sipped seemed to claw its way down my throat as I began to wonder why in the world was I here. Was making a speech important enough for me to go through this pain? Was this some kind of rite of passage for community acceptance?

As I sat at the head table among some of the who's who in the city, the protagonist in Ralph Ellison's *Invisible Man* eased into my thoughts as if he had been summoned. Perhaps he had been. He had been forced to make a speech before the town's leading white citizens after he had been beaten in a fight. With his mouth filled with blood, his lips swollen like an inner tube, and perspiration streaming down his bruised body, he was determined to speak in order to convince the crowd of his superior intelligence. Was this me? Did I, too, have something to prove?

As I think about it now, whatever the motives, my need to deliver that speech was the beginning of my determination not to succumb to the fear, anger, pain and loneliness of being unwell. It was also the beginning of my refusal to see myself as sick.

In the midst of silverware scraping against plates and cups clanging against saucers, I began to speak. With the tissue in my hand, I was ready for any embarrassing moments. The surgery had changed the sound of my voice, and I struggled to hear myself as I spoke about the obligation of teachers, leaders, and other persons of responsibility to try to live according to Psalms 51, Verse 10.

"Give me a clean heart, O God, and renew a right spirit within me" bubbled from my mouth as I connected the scripture to meeting community needs. Again, my mouth filled with saliva during my garbling "group development" and "ethnic solidarity" in the same sentence. Quickly, I ran a tissue over my lips, cleared my throat, and continued competing with the buzzing, humming, clinking and clanking of the crowd.

I concluded to a standing ovation, but I thought most of the audience had been rude, noisy, unappreciative, and ignorant. I probably exaggerated their behavior, but it didn't help matters when my efforts turned out to be *gratis*, not that I truly expected to be compensated. I did wonder, however, why I didn't negotiate the terms before I agreed to participate. Perhaps my negligence reflected what I had begun to refer to as the invisible woman syndrome—doing too much for too little. I left the banquet with a sore throat and a bitter taste in my mouth.

A few days later, I received a dozen red roses and a note of thanks from the activist who had invited me to speak for the occasion. Without thinking, my hand found its way to my throat and I swallowed with severe difficulty. This was my reward for a night of pain.

I sat the roses on the table and bent to inhale their fragrance. There was none.

Chapter 3

OMINOUS NEWS

The next week I kept my appointment with the ENT specialist, who was prepared to give me the results of the pathology report from the biopsy. I had papillary carcinoma, a form of thyroid cancer—not the worst, but certainly something to be concerned about. In his reserved way, he told me it was best to have my thyroid removed in about two weeks.

A few days later, I developed pain in my side, resulting in my family doctor's ordering an ultrasound.

On Thursday before the test, my doctor called to tell me I also needed to see a vascular surgeon to discuss putting in a dialysis access. She gave me a long strange foreign-sounding name and told me to contact the surgeon immediately. Following the thyroid biopsy, my creatinine had increased from an average of 5 to 7.2, numbers that meant not only did I have to deal with thyroid cancer, my kidneys were now showing signs of impending failure.

I looked at the paper on which I had scribbled the name. "Oh, Jesus, who is this doctor you mentioned?"

"A vascular surgeon. You'll like him."

"How soon should I call?"

"Today. You need to take care of this as soon as possible."

"But, I'm going to see my uncle this weekend in Philadelphia."

"No, don't make that trip." She was more adamant than I had ever heard her.

"But, . . ."

"No, I am very much opposed to your going out of town. It's definitely not a good idea."

"But my uncle just turned 91, and I want to visit him."

"Well," she said, returning to her usually delicate voice. "I'm sure he will understand the circumstances and want you to stay home. I insist."

I had never heard her insist on anything and I was somewhat shocked. Actually, it frightened me.

"Now call the vascular surgeon and make an appointment for the dialysis access. You need to do that."

"But . . . why do I need to call him now? Am I going on dialysis now? Why can't I make the trip?"

"I just don't want you away from home . . . not now. I mean you could be in Philadelphia and something could happen. Let's just say your kidneys failed and you were way up there with none of your doctors . . . I just think that's too big a risk. I'm really opposed to any such trip," she said again . She repeated the number of the vascular surgeon and emphatically encouraged me to give him a call. "You need that access; I don't know how else to say it."

"What's this access going to be like?" I asked, trying to recover from the disappointment of not being able to make the trip. "I mean, what are we talking about?"

"He'll probably put a catheter in your neck."

"What?" Astounded, I squeezed the receiver. "In my neck?" I fingered my neck. "Oh no!" I shook my head adamantly. "I can't deal with that! I can't be walking around with a tube sticking from my neck." I realized I was almost shouting and tried to calm down.

"Aw, it won't be that bad. There'll be no stress on the thyroid area. They'll just find a vein and insert the catheter. You can wear a scarf and nobody will be able to see it. It'll be all right, I promise."

I didn't want to ask any more questions, since I had already held her on the phone longer than she probably anticipated when she called me. Besides, what else could I say?

"No Philadelphia," she repeated. "Okay?"

I hung up the phone and fell into a chair at the kitchen table. None of this seemed natural to me. It was as if I were caught up in some kind of whirlwind of bad luck and snatched along, jerked this way and that, and what was even worse, I had no control over anything. How was I going to deal with this tube protruding from my neck? I just couldn't do it. I wouldn't. And now, I couldn't even make the trip to Philadelphia because my doctor had put the fear of God in me. Moreover, I would have to spend the weekend alone, since my husband was on a business trip and would not return until the following week.

I called my uncle to tell him about my change of plans. I didn't give him all the dismal details, but I told him enough about my health concerns that he agreed it wouldn't be wise to make the trip. Then, my cousin, who had also been looking forward to my visit, called me for all the information he knew I didn't tell my uncle. I think he was the first person to whom I admitted my fear. Surprisingly, this acknowledgement provided a kind of freedom from the inherited notion I needed to be strong in the face of struggle. I was not only tired, I was weak and weary, and for once I wasn't ashamed of it.

That weekend, my cousin flew to Cincinnati to spend Saturday and Sunday with me. While he was here, we talked openly about the thyroid cancer and my dread at being hooked to a machine to stay alive. I told him about my dream of walking the street with a tube protruding from my neck like some kind of space monster, frightening children and sending them fleeing to their parents.

Acknowledging a certain amount of vanity, I also talked freely about growing older and the trepidation brought on by declining health. "When you were younger, did you ever think about getting older and developing some kind of chronic illness?" I asked as we sat on the deck, feeling the delicate wind that bathed our faces.

"No." He sipped his drink. "And besides, you're not old. I'm ten years your senior and I don't see myself as old."

"Yeah, but you haven't been diagnosed with anything. I think this thyroid cancer and kidney problem have made me think more about getting older. I wonder if this is all happening because it's just time."

"What do you mean?" He leaned closer to me.

"You know, I am older. Some people claim they don't pay attention to their age."

"Bull!" He set his drink on the table. "I don't believe that. Once you're past forty, little things begin to happen, like a pull here and a strain there. And I believe it happens to everybody, but it doesn't always mean 'old' in the sense that the West looks at old. I mean it doesn't necessarily say you're on your way to the grave. It just means you're closer to it. But you do notice it. You might not say anything, but you notice it. And then, you know, there are those times I see a woman and I hold my stomach in until she's out of view."

We laughed.

"Well, with women, it's tougher and I don't need to recite to you all the things people say about women getting older, especially older and sickly."

"Yeah, I guess you're right. All those commercials about Depends, stuff to hold your dentures in place, and . . . "

"And yeah, pills for hot flashes."

DUCK SUMMER: *MY ODYSSEY AS A DIALYSIS PATIENT*

Our conversations gave me the chance to laugh at myself and notice the enchanting early summer weather with the sweet smell of lilac and jasmine in the air. Trying not to be overwhelmed by thoughts of illnesses, we took every available opportunity to embrace the outdoors. Downtown we watched the crowds frolic in the warm afternoon promises of summer, and listened to the muffled chatter of small children apparently lined up for a program on the skywalk.

For a late afternoon lunch, we ate outside under a colorful umbrella, sharing conversation and laughter. Occasionally we were quiet, concentrating on the distant tune of a tenor sax that must have come from inside the restaurant. Soon John Coltrane and Johnny Hartman threaded the air with tunes from their 1963 album.

"I'm going to go home and pull out that CD," I said. "I need to hear that again."

"What do you know about Coltrane and Hartman?"

"A lot." I folded my arms and sighed. "I know their music will bring you out of the doldrums and make you think anything is possible. It's just that beautiful."

I leaned back in the chair and relaxed to the melodious winds of Coltrane. I was alive and a part of everything that was going on around me. For a while, I didn't think of myself as the one with thyroid cancer and looming kidney failure. I was only one of the many, and I delighted in it. How long had it been since I savored the beauty of this world with its sounds and sights and smells? Why did it take a scare for me to see, listen, and hear all the beauty around me?

Though I had a trouble-free weekend, one where I packed my problems in a trunk and pushed it to the back of my closet, the trouble was not gone forever. The next week I went to see the vascular surgeon, an Indian, who explained to me the particulars of the access procedure. I entered his office with a negative attitude. My eyes, I know, were pulled together in an intimidating frown, my mouth turned down at the corners. I was ready to strike out with the least provocation. With all the advancements in medicine, I was downgraded to having this primitive looking thing sticking from my neck. There was no way I was going to have a stupid tube protruding from my neck.

"Well," he said, overlooking my sarcasm. "You don't have to do anything you don't want to do. But your doctor says you need this."

"I'm not on dialysis yet."

"Yes, but according to my information, you will be, and pretty soon." He was a gentle-sounding man, dark, with compassionate eyes that said much more than he did.

"I don't want some *thing* sticking from my neck."

"What thing?"

"The tube."

"There's not going to be any tube sticking from your neck. Where'd you get that little piece of information?" He stretched his eyes in jest. It will be in your chest. Hidden."

"Oh." I was embarrassed. "But I thought . . ." I knew vanity was one of my problems, but I was about to become a lunatic over this whole thing.

"We don't do that unless we can't get the access into the chest or it's an emergency. You're getting yours ahead of time, so everything is okay."

*****

On the day of the access surgery, I learned the ultrasound of my stomach had shown nothing, which meant that I had one less thing to worry about as I prepared for the procedure. Having done all the usual pre-admission testing, I assumed I would get the usual dose of anesthesia, but instead they injected a local anesthetic, which didn't seem to have any more effect than a couple of Tylenol. When they rolled me into the pale green room with the big, bright glaring light, I was fully conscious. In fact, I was still awake and alert when the surgeon made a quarter inch incision in my upper chest and ran a small tube into my skin. I could feel the tube moving inside my body, then a clawing, low inside my throat choking me, giving me the urge to swallow.

"It hurts; it hurts," I mumbled through congestion.

"Hold on. Hold on. We're almost finished." The surgeon put down his instrument and ordered a chest x-ray to see if the catheter were in the right position.

"Looks good," he said, as I was becoming drowsy.

After all the probing and pushing, I finally drifted off to sleep. When I awakened, I felt the heavy bandages plastered around my neck. I let my hand slide up the left side of my chest and found a little tube about four inches long with a small rectangular capping. I prayed I would never have to use this thing called a "tesio catheter."

After the surgery for the dialysis access, the hospital put me into a room with a woman who had undergone thyroid surgery a couple of days earlier. Overweight and obviously still fatigued from her surgery, she didn't talk very much; the T. V. talked for her. It was as loud as if she were listening to it from across the hall. Frequently, her daughter came to visit, each time bringing some kind of fast food —fries, burgers, muffins, and a big soft drink, which her mother consumed with such passion and vigor I wondered what it must feel like to enjoy something that much. I was baffled that she could swallow so soon after the surgery, but I assumed her problem must have been different from the thyroid procedure I had undergone.

Just before I was scheduled for dismissal, the same doctor who had performed the biopsy and removed half of my thyroid, came into the room to give my roommate the results from her surgery. There was no cancer. I heard her breathe a sigh of relief and although I was glad for her, I couldn't help but wonder why I was picked for the thyroid cancer *and* kidney failure? Was there some kind of connection? Or, did God just look down from Heaven and casually say, "I think I'll give both to her this time?" How does God make these decisions? Is it God's decision? My questions about God didn't cease over the next few weeks, and the next thing I knew I was undergoing surgery on the remaining part of my thyroid in case there were any leftover cancer cells. Was I doing some kind of penance for me, or perhaps someone who had come before me? For whose sins was I atoning?

When I awakened from this second surgery, I sensed God's presence. A sense of ease and comfort surrounded me, even though my throat was in dire pain and I could barely breathe. With the slightest inhale and exhale, I screamed inside myself, but somehow the soreness didn't connect to my state of being. Calm and at peace, I lay as if there were no earth and no sky, and my body simply gave way to space.

In this stage, I learned there were no residual cancer cells, but the surgeon removed the remaining part of thyroid anyway.

The serenity I felt after the surgery eventually faded, and a renewed sense of fear and uncertainty emerged; the most profound was whether or not my creatinine had risen after the second thyroid surgery. Fortunately, the level didn't change, and I remained free of the dialysis machine. Other than having to talk to an endocrinologist to schedule follow-up care, I was dismissed from the hospital after a couple of days.

Between the last week of May and the first few days of July, I had undergone several kidney and thyroid diagnostic and pre-op tests, three surgeries and one biopsy. Caught up in a whirlwind of medical tests, doctors, nurses, technicians, and operating rooms, I had wandered through a world of hospital green. Scared most of the time, I had become part of a game I didn't understand, and the other players seemed to be having fun at my expense. I decided it must have been a test—endurance, patience, perhaps strength. There had to be a reason why all of these things were happening to me, especially in such close proximity. Otherwise, I was certainly caught up in some kind of Kafkaesque nightmare.

But I couldn't wake myself. Nor could I escape the memories and fears of the thyroidectomy, catheter, creatinine number, postponed trip to Philadelphia, swollen ankles, and unimaginable fatigue. Everything was always with me, and I began to wonder if there would ever come a time when I could relax with a sense that I had regained some control over my life. Often, my nerves were frayed and the least little annoyance—cloudy weather, litter in my yard, or the ring of the telephone—sent me into a rage where I could feel my pulse beating in my neck and my heart racing. When would all of this end?

Chapter 4

IN SEARCH OF GOD

Wandering through the unforgiving maze of hospitals, doctors, laboratories, and diagnoses, I began to question my faith. Unlike childhood, when I could feel the direct involvement of God in my life, I couldn't sense His presence now.

When I was around seven or eight, I dreamed a wall was creeping from the sky, shutting out the sunshine and shielding me in darkness. Frightened and bewildered, I called on God, and almost immediately, the ominous wall receded and a promising sun appeared. I took this enigmatic vision as a sign God would always save me; certainly, He would take care of this papillary carcinoma. But when the cancer didn't just vanish, and my case was turned over to an endocrinologist, I assumed God decided He needed to steal away for a while.

So I went looking for Him. Not the God of the spiritually gifted, who claim a kind of metaphysical connection to Him, but the burning bush God, the God of Abraham, who delivered the Israelites from bondage and parted the Red Sea—the God who showed me the light when I was a child. I needed the sympathetic God, who sent his son, part human and part divine, to raise Lazarus from the dead, to cast out the demons, to restore health to the sick and sight to the blind. I wanted to hear His voice, to grasp His hand, and realize His presence.

In my quest to find God, I rededicated myself to my church, put mind and heart in my membership, and became an integral part. Still, I was uncertain about achieving the spiritual revival I was seeking.

I remember a Bible Study series where the minister questioned the group about how we experienced God. About fifteen of us sat around a table listening to her suggest ways we might identify God's presence in our lives, and the more she talked, the more spiritual distance I recognized between God and me. When it was my time to testify, I suddenly heard my voice pouring through tears I couldn't control or explain. "I am trying to establish some relationship with God, but it just seems I am now going through a dry spell. I'm crawling through the desert," I remember saying. "I'm digging my knees into the sand, sniffing the dry dust, and yet trying to make it through. Actually, I'm trying to *find* God."

"What makes you think He's not right here with you?" She chuckled. Have you been still long enough to hear Him? You know what He said?" Her voice became firm. "Be still and know that I am God."

After class, I turned Pastor Verra Gales's comments over in my mind. Perhaps it was not God I was searching for, but faith enough to believe He would see me through my health crises. Maybe I already had the necessary faith—the mustard-seed size Jesus speaks of in the New Testament, but I couldn't sense it or feel it.

My quest for a stronger faith led me to such books as Peter Gomes, *The Good Book*, James Melvin's *Conversations with God*, Harold S. Kushner's *When Bad Things Happen to Good People*, and the Bible. While these books broadened my perspective on religious questions, none of them revitalized the stubbornly waning faith so characteristic of this period of my life. Gomes' discussion of the Bible's position on controversial issues, such as difference, sexual preference and the like, Melvin's portrayal of the Black Christian experience as reflected in prayer, and Kushner's interesting position on the role of nature and fate in life's trials, presented a mosaic of challenging ideas, but none of them showed me how to strengthen my faith. When I turned to the Bible, I did so with the knowledge that the answer lay somewhere in its many pages, but as the old folks used to say, a vague understanding of scripture obscures the questions and the answers.

This faith dilemma was consuming me. With all my medical

troubles, I concentrated on nothing more than my struggle to embrace that rudimentary conviction I learned as a child. I couldn't understand why, if I had any kind of relationship with God at all, He wouldn't heal me. I prayed constantly, asking Him to strengthen me in my weaker moments and to help me to find the faith that seemed so elusive to me now.

Still, I felt as if I were trapped in the turbulence of one of life's worst storms and the debris was crushing me. Was I being punished for something? Did I have some kind of debt to pay for some family indiscretion? Did I deserve what was happening to me? Do we get what we deserve?

Exploring the subject of getting what we deserve proved to be a daunting task. If I took the position that we do, then I had to be prepared to accept all the tragedy that transpires in people's lives as recompense for past behavior, a position I couldn't accept. People experience all forms of misfortune—hunger, poverty, natural disasters, illnesses, and some of the same people spend their lives working for the good. Children, too young to discern right from wrong, go to bed hungry every night, experience unimaginable illnesses, die in wars, and yet have done nothing to warrant such horrors. People don't always get what they deserve, I concluded, and they don't always deserve what they get. If life could be explained in such simple terms, perhaps we could understand the inconsistencies, contradictions, absurdities and even the unfairness that too often accompanies day-to-day living.

It was not very long before I came to understand that if I didn't want to become a victim of my own obsessions, I had to face some truths about myself. First, I was taking myself much too seriously. Self-pity had come without warning, jumped into my arms, and been nursed like a baby. It had drunk the milk of acceptance and flourished like a well-nurtured child. I let it become my progeny.

Second, with all the difficulties confronting many of those

around me, I started to wonder what made me think I should be exempt. On one occasion, when I had to take more tests at the hospital, I found the lobby filled with disabled people, including children, teenagers, and old people, moving around in wheelchairs. One woman, fortyish, pushed herself with one leg, while the other leg, amputated just below the knee, was folded under her hip. A teen-aged boy sat curled in his chair, his head bouncing aimlessly towards his chest, his gnarled fingers fanning the air.

And here I sat, having whined for weeks because things weren't going my way. I blamed God for my troubles because He was the only one who could change things. I questioned my faith because praying didn't bring me what I wanted. If I were faithful, I thought, God would do what I asked. Conversely, since God had allowed my struggles to continue, I must be unfaithful. I was responding as if God answered prayers based solely on the level of the petitioner's faith.

I shared my inner struggles with some of my friends because I was still looking for answers and clarity. One friend reminded me of the well-known story of the man who learned that the torrential rains in his area would eventually result in a flood and he should evacuate his home. The man refused, declaring he would wait on God because God would save him. When the water reached the porch, an SUV came by, but the man ignored it, as he did the rowboat appearing after the water got to the second story. By the time the water was at the roof, a helicopter came to rescue him, but the man waved it on, as he was still waiting for God. When he was swallowed by flood and went to Heaven, he asked God why He didn't save him, to which God replied, "I sent an SUV, a boat, and a helicopter. Why didn't you get on one of them?"

I had been too self-absorbed to recognize the "vehicles" God had sent to save me from the storm. Good medical care, insurance, supportive family and friends, and a thorough family physician, who had the vision and the patience to detect a problem in my neck. In all of my weaknesses and doubts, my questions of faith and my lack of spiritual clarity, God had been with me all along. Grappling with my health problems and my relationship with Him, I realized I was gaining spiritual empowerment through a developing awareness about God and the many ways He reveals Himself.

Had it not been for the confrontation with my perceived faithlessness and the subsequent clarity of thought and vision, I would scarcely have been able to greet my family, who at the insistence of my mother, decided to pay me a visit. I had planned not to divulge anything health-related to them, but my mother could tell in the sound of my voice that something was wrong. Apparently unconvinced when I told her I had undergone minor surgery, which revealed only a cyst on my tonsils, she constantly reminded me to keep an eye on it because I wouldn't want it to develop into something "worse."

Though my mother was the brave one, I knew this was not the time to say anything about thyroid cancer to her or my sister and brother. All they would be able to hear was "cancer," and I didn't want to see the fear in their eyes, nor hear the strain in their voices as they tried to think of people who had survived a similar "condition". (To them, cancer was a condition). Moreover, since I didn't have the energy to combat their anxieties, it was preferable to weave a more acceptable explanation for my illness.

My family stayed with me three days, and each day I folded more into myself because I couldn't bear lying and pretending that even something as commonplace as breathing was not causing me unbearable pain.

It took a few weeks before the soreness in my throat dwindled to a slight tickle. But my thyroid treatment was far from over. After the second surgical procedure, my case was turned over to an endocrinologist who began his course of treatment by prescribing Cytomel, a drug designed to strip the body of iodine and prepare me for the succeeding radioactive therapy. Even though I didn't have to undergo the typical chemotherapy, the post-operative procedures were assuredly not without distress.

My energy level had declined severely and I dragged myself from one site to another, searching for a resting place. Although the doctor said nothing about the effects of the medicine on energy, I made the erroneous assumption that Cytomel was an antidote for the sluggishness resulting from the thyroidectomy. I took the Cytomel for six weeks, becoming weaker by the day, but taking solace in the idea that the medicine was preparing me for the final stage of my treatment.

During these Cytomel weeks, I flew to a place I found advertised in a magazine, Jekyll Island, Georgia, where I tried to put the previous weeks behind me. A beautiful island on the southern coast of Georgia, Jekyll is one of Georgia's state-owned vacation resorts, and as such, had not become the prey of developers. In this quiet, sparsely populated area of enchanting beauty, oak trees webbed in Spanish moss tower over each side of the winding roads, forming an arch sheltering the thin traffic. Hide-a-way cottages tucked behind mimosa trees and palmettos stand against a cloudless sky. The soft wind singing over the Atlantic kindles the imagination, and watching the morning sun peep over the ocean is like seeing the face of God.

I marvel now that I was able to engage in several physical activities at Jekyll Island, despite my almost complete lack of energy. Mesmerized by the local splendor, I must have stepped outside of my frail body and took on a frame strong enough to embrace the region. I biked, rode horses, walked along the beach and through the woods, and wandered about Jekyll's historic district, the setting of the mansions of late 19th century industrialists such as J. P. Morgan, Goodyear, and others who once owned the island and a vast number of people like me.

I visualized lazy women in corseted dresses, sitting under oak trees, sipping mint tea, while men, clustered like grapes, boasted through cigar smoke of the rise in their stocks or the performance of a new race horse. Black women, scurrying about the kitchen, frequently glanced at the clock to make sure the privileged little ones, industrialists-to-be, would get their mid-day meal in time for their afternoon nap. A little brown boy or girl shaded an old white couple with a large palmetto. Far away from the mansions, black men maintained the knock-knock rhythm of building the latest guesthouse, tavern, or slave hut.

 Passing the few cottages shared by more than two-dozen servants, I imagined them cramped in their quarters at night, or leaning against an arthritic oak tree taking in the tranquil darkness before the next day's work. Walking through their meagerly furnished dwellings, I sensed their presence all around me, their voices beckoning me to remember that they and I are kin.

 If it were possible to escape the things that happened that summer, Jekyll Island would have been the ideal place to do it. However, as I wandered over one of the most idyllic settings I have ever seen, the world of medicine and health care was always somewhere in the back of my mind, nudging and nagging me. The tesio catheter was still in my chest, and eventually I could rarely summon the alter ego to ride a horse or pedal a bike. When I tried to run along the beach, my legs seemed tied to bags of wet sand. Even walking drained me.

 I no longer had the energy to get into the water and I knew that even the puniest wave would knock me into the ocean. On those days when I braved the beach, I dragged my chair along the sand and flopped, determined to read the books and magazines I had brought with me. Sitting there, however, listening to the thrashing of the waves, my hands dropped to the sides of the chair while my book slid between my legs, its pages flapping against the ocean breeze.

 I had done some reading on the Internet about the thyroid and extreme fatigue, and I also had a bookbag of material from the hospital.

DUCK SUMMER: *MY ODYSSEY AS A DIALYSIS PATIENT*

Based on the information, I now assumed my fatigue was the result of the thyroidectomy and later the medication. Therefore, when I returned to Cincinnati, I went immediately to my endocrinologist to inform him that my dosage of thyroid medicine was insufficient. I explained my symptoms, telling him that I knew I should be feeling more like myself. He looked at me sympathetically and said, "Well, I doubt it's all due to the medicine. You're functioning on almost no kidney, and that's probably what it is."

Still unwilling to believe I was approaching dialysis, I ignored his comment and vowed to revise my exercise program to enhance my energy level. God would do the rest.

The next week I saw my kidney doctor, who said things were not looking the way he had hoped. Though the BUN and creatinine still had not climbed any higher than they had after the second thyroid surgery, the numbers were still lingering near the danger zone. He didn't recommend dialysis at that particular visit, but instead, wrote an order for me to go to the hospital to have my catheter flushed . . . just in case. "No need to take chances," he warned.

When I went to the dialysis unit at the hospital to have the catheter flushed, I stepped into a nightmare. On one side of a big pale green room, there were eight dialysis machines, big 1950's computer-looking clanging contraptions. On the other side were eight more, each facing the other. The nurse's station was in the next room behind a partition, across from which were two smaller rooms, one with six dialysis machines and another with two. In all, there must have been about twenty four dialysis machines and a person connected to each one.

For more than twenty-five years, I had known about my chronic kidney disease. However, I had never even allowed myself to imagine what a kidney machine looked like, and I certainly refused to go to the hospital or clinic to look at one. Why should I? What did it mean to me? I had never thought much about the people who, I learned, had to be hooked to these machines at least three times a week for three to five hours. All of this was a part of the general health care system; it was not a part of me.

Things had apparently changed, though, since here I was, standing in the dialysis section of the hospital, listening to the discordant beeping of the machines and watching dialysis patients. I had stepped into a mechanical medical hell.

What was even more unnerving was the condition of the people hooked to these machines. Sick people were everywhere. It didn't occur to me then that a hospital unit would have more sick people on dialysis than the free standing clinics. Looking around the pale green alcohol-smelling room and waiting for the nurse to flush my catheter, I felt warm tears creep down my cheeks and connect under my chin. Patients with one arm or one leg missing and even a few with no legs lay sprawled on gurneys, tubes running to and from their bodies. Some were in wheel chairs; some on stretchers, and a few appeared to be independent. I watched a technician raise a woman from a stretcher so she could throw up. She couldn't even wipe her mouth.

I had been so engrossed in the robotic surroundings I had not noticed that many of the patients attached to these machines were Black, while most of the nurses, technicians, and other healthcare professionals were white. Were black people the primary victims of renal failure? There was a look of resignation on the patients' faces and whether they were nodding, completely asleep or half watching the television attached to the wall at each dialysis station, they appeared to have submitted themselves to the machine. They were all breathing, but there seemed to be no life.

Was this going to be me in a few weeks? A few months? Was this what my life would be like if I went on dialysis? *When* I went on dialysis? Would I be unable to take care of myself? Would they have to bring me in on a stretcher? Would I be in a wheel chair? Would I be able to work? Would I be sick all the time? The questions kept coming, and while I listened to the beeping machines, I realized how afraid I was of the impending changes in my life.

The appointment at the dialysis unit was a long nightmare, where nurses in green pants and tops moved in slow motion, and technicians, manipulating icons on the machines' computers, also appeared to move in dreamlike fashion. I became an invalid. The patients were steeled like zombies as unclean blood flowed from their veins into the tube, circulated through the machine for filtering, and returned clean to their body. This was life to them; it was death to me.

I stood paralyzed until the head nurse came towards me, calling my name and snapping me out of my trance. "Ms. Hall, we need to take a look at that catheter'."

Nervously, I unbuttoned my blouse and flipped out the catheter from my chest.

The nurse lifted its triangular end, inserted a needle of heparin and pumped. Nothing happened. She grimaced and tried again.

Still nothing.

"Oomph," she grunted, pursing her lips and shaking her head. "It's clotted. There's nothing you can do with that. It's no good now." She withdrew the needle.

"Suppose I need it?" I wiped perspiration from my forehead with the back of my hand. A hot flash cooked my insides.

"You can't use this one," she said as if a clotted catheter were commonplace. "You'll just have to get another one. Let's just hope you won't ever have to use it." She turned and walked away to get another catheter.

When I left the dialysis unit with a new catheter, I told myself

I would never come here again. This was not going to happen to me. God would not allow it.

Chapter 5

SEAGULLS AND ITALIAN ICE

A couple of weeks after the trip to the hospital dialysis unit, I had an appointment with a registered licensed dietician, adding yet another step to what seemed to be an endless treatment for thyroid cancer. After completing the Cytomel, the doctor prescribed a ten-day non-iodine diet, as a major part of the preparation for the radioactive therapy. The hospital dietician, who spoke with a heavy Middle Eastern accent, informed me of all the diet restrictions on the non-iodine diet. Much more limiting than a simple no-salt diet, the non-iodine regiment allowed absolutely nothing with iodine or salt, which meant that anything I consumed would taste like paper. The objective of this kind of diet is to eliminate as much iodine from my body as possible before the scans and the treatment with radioactive iodine.

Since I had about two weeks before I was scheduled to begin the low iodine diet, and I didn't want to waste the in-between time besieged by dread, I decided this would be a good time for a trip to the east coast. My husband and I wanted to go to Delaware to visit his parents. It would give us another chance to spend some time at the ocean while we shared a holiday with family. Moreover, I could use the trip to pretend there was nothing unusual going on in my life.

I tried again to put the intractable thyroid situation into an inactive mental file, but the fact that I still had more therapy to undergo before the summer was over rendered this an impossible feat. Then there was also the catheter dangling from my chest, which battled with my thyroidectomy for attention and made me aware that no matter how hard I tried, I couldn't think away my health challenges.

For a brief while, though, the east coast was an untroubled spot, and like Jekyll Island, Georgia, a place of peace and contentment. The fresh water breeze blowing in from the Delaware River, delicious food, haunting sea gulls flying over the marsh, and always the distant sound of river traffic, reminded me of more innocent and uncomplicated times. Watching the fisherman wrestle with buckets of crab and fish carried me back to childhood summers in Philadelphia when my uncle let the top down on his 1957 Chevy and drove to Atlantic City. The tiny glittering souvenirs on vendor stands along the boardwalk, the sweet salty smell of taffy, and the distant slapping of the beach by the low tide, are all with me now. I can still taste the cotton candy and laugh at the pictures we took in the $2 photography booths.

In more recent times, one of the greatest joys of summers in Delaware was the long walks from Jefferson Farms, a suburban area of Wilmington, to New Castle's historic district, preserved from Colonial times. I looked forward to the familiar trek past the houses along the highway onto the tree-shaded street leading to the center of New Castle. A five-mile jaunt from Jefferson Farms, through the historic district and the park to the edge of the Delaware River, the trip is filled with the sounds and smells of the river and the marsh. Wrapped in the misty breeze, I often gazed at the sea gulls as they flapped their wings against the soft wind. Ducks floated easily over small streams, and I could never understand how they hid their death defying struggle to float calmly along. The sky appeared to hang low enough for me to touch, and the sun's rays gleamed on the river water and the nearby creeks.

When I reached the park benches, exhausted and drymouthed, I wasn't sure I could go any further. I bought an Italian Ice cone from one of the concession stands, and found a bench a few feet from the river's edge. Watching people throw peanuts at the sea gulls and ducks, I bit into the Italian Ice, letting the ice chips cool the inside of my mouth and trickle down my throat. Of the many times I had made this excursion, I couldn't remember ever being as exhausted. It was as if I carried a 50-pound load the entire distance. I leaned against the bench, trying to catch my breath, as my clothes clung to my damp body. The sea gulls danced over the water, still flapping their wings and squawking as they formed a random pattern against the sky. Finally, I guzzled the juice left from my melting ice and mentally prepared myself for the journey home.

Slowly walking back, I envisioned lying down in the field along the highway and resting in the tall green weeds. Tired and drained, I assumed the problem was my lack of sleep the last few days and the rush to make the trip as scheduled. Anyway, out of nowhere, on the last half mile of the walk, I began to get a second wind, which renewed my sense of wellbeing and gave me the confidence that everything was, in fact, all right.

The next day I was as wiped out as I was at the river, but I forced myself to go along with family plans. That night, we all went to dinner at one of Delaware's most popular seafood restaurants. Instead of eating more seafood than I should, the way I usually do, I stood before the raw bar gazing at the oysters and watching the lemon slices blur against the leaf lettuce. Back at the table, I picked over the food as if it were rancid. It was only the *memory* of the taste of crab cakes and lobster tails that encouraged me to attempt to eat. I simply had no appetite. I nibbled on small pieces of lettuce, pushed cubes of tomato and carrot strips from one place to another on my plate, and finally waved for the waitress to come and take it away.

Watching the rest of the family enjoy their food, I decided to try some pasta salad, since I thought pasta might be easier on the stomach. Shortly after the first bite, I felt a small pocket of immovable gas in the right side of my stomach. Without drawing attention to myself, I massaged my stomach and wondered if this were the beginning of one of those two to three-day bouts with gas that had so often sent me to the emergency room. For the remainder of the time we spent at the restaurant, the gas didn't dissipate; it just knotted in my side, moved to my upper intestines, and finally took on the feel of a big jagged-edged rock.

When we reached home, I gulped two Rolaids and lay on the bed. The two white pasty pills had no effect on the gas; in fact, what was gas had now become an annoying stomach ache, characterized by both bloating and pain. As the night progressed, I thrashed about with stomach cramps that became almost unbearable. I tried to find a comfortable position from which I could rest and eventually fall asleep, but both rest and sleep eluded me. The only way I could bear the pain was to lie between my left side and stomach, a position that had my face practically buried in the mattress.

By morning, I was not only suffering from the gas pains that exploded throughout my stomach and back during the night, I was sore from my rib cage to my lower stomach from wrestling with the gas. There was no way I would be able to go downstairs, and therefore, with the exception of trips to the bathroom, I spent the entire day in bed.

My aunts came to my sick bed bringing toast, tea and prayers. I took a few sips of tea, and since I knew they would not leave me alone until I ate the toast, I forced down a couple of bites. Knowing we were supposed to fly back to Cincinnati Monday morning, I tried to sit up long enough to prove I could make the trip. Both my husband and mother-in-law insisted they take me to the emergency room, but I pleaded with them to hold off because I knew it would be an insurance nightmare.

By the middle of Sunday afternoon, I was praying that Monday morning would find me able to get on a plane and fly back to Cincinnati. I was as ill as ever, and I knew if I looked as badly as I felt, the airline personnel would never let me board the plane.

On Monday morning, I went to God, this time asking for the strength to get on the plane and stay alert at least until I could get home. Conscious that any slight movement would send me into a frenzy of pain, I dragged myself slowly out of bed for the first time since

Saturday, got dressed and prepared for the car ride to the Philadelphia airport. By now the agony had become its own person.

By the time we arrived in Cincinnati, everything between my rib cage and my pelvic area knotted, and gas bubbles stomped from my stomach to my back. Unlike before, when the nurses and physicians checked to make sure I wasn't having a heart attack, I decided to avoid a trip to the hospital and take another wait-and-see night. I really didn't have the energy for the ride, the hospital wait, or the physician's probing.

On Monday, after suffering all night and despite my daughter's insistence that I call my internist, I phoned the gastroenterologist, since this was clearly a digestive problem. The gastroenterologist had become one of a group of physicians recommended by my internist over the years. As my regular gastroenterologist was unavailable, (as to be expected given the way things were going), I was assigned to an assistant, a good enough physician, I suppose, but one I had never seen before. After taking my pulse and blood pressure, the doctor pressed on my stomach a couple of times, and prescribed some antacids, which I took Monday night, Tuesday, and Wednesday.

The pills only eased the gas pains. I was still sick with no appetite and now, absolutely no energy. By late afternoon on Wednesday, I had become nauseated and couldn't even keep down water. Ordinarily, I could get rid of the gas pains in a day or a day and a night, but this time they had already lasted five days. It was time to call the internist. The nausea was a new and more frightening symptom of something I didn't understand.

"How long have you been nauseated?" She asked after we talked about the gas pains.

"It started today, shortly after noon."

"Well," she said. "Let's get you to the emergency room and rule out kidney failure."

"Kidney failure? It couldn't be that." Suddenly I felt as if I were about to faint. "But . . . But, I'm urinating as usual." Kidney failure had not crossed my mind. It couldn't be happening now. Not now. I wasn't ready yet.

"Yeah, but that won't make a difference now. We should check out the kidneys before we go any further."

I hadn't been at the hospital more than twenty minutes before they were rolling me in and taking blood, after which an ER physician ordered a pain pill. Just as the gas pains were subsiding, allowing me to rest for the first time in five days, the doctor returned, gazing at his chart. "I'm afraid it's kidney failure. The nurse is getting in touch with the doctor."

"Are you sure?" I rose from the stretcher, realizing for the first time in days that my stomach wasn't hurting.

"Yes," he said, sucking his bottom lip and shaking his head. "Your creatinine is 9 and your BUN is over 90."

Since a healthy creatinine is somewhere between .5 and 1.5 and a BUN shouldn't be over 10 or 12, I knew I was in trouble. My kidneys had failed.

That night my internist admitted me to the hospital and the next morning, a nurse wheeled me into the operating room where women and men in pale green uniforms prepared me for the insertion of another catheter. Because they didn't administer general anesthesia, I was conscious during most of the procedure. The physicians numbed the area where they inserted the catheter, but they had to place the extended tube in a specific area in order for me to receive dialysis appropriately. Again, I could feel the tube traveling through my chest, restricting my breathing and giving me a choking sensation. After a while, a nurse rolled in an x-ray machine, and the physician checked to see if the catheter was accurately placed.

Everything was okay. It was almost time for what the doctors had predicted twenty-five years earlier—dialysis or "the D word," which is how many with ESRD (End Stage Renal Disease) often referred to dialysis.

*****

And so it was. After twenty-five years, it had finally come to pass. I had gone into kidney failure, and that afternoon, shortly after 12, on September 4, 1998, I underwent my first dialysis treatment.

Chapter 6

THE HOSPITAL MAZE

The dialysis procedure wasn't new to me since I had been gathering information on it for years, but I still didn't know what the actual patient experience would be like. The machine, with the transparent tubes, the red and green flashing signals, and the filtering instrument, called the artificial "kidney," had all been something I *might* come to know one day, *if* my kidneys failed. They had now failed and these machines and tubes had become an integral part of my life.

My initial treatment was in the hospital.

The nurse hooked two tubes to my catheter. One pumped the blood from the catheter into the bloodline. After which she added Heparin, a blood thinner, to prevent clotting. Blood flowed into the dialyzer which, filtered it of excess fluid, waste and salt. The other tube returned the filtered blood to my heart, which pumped it throughout my body. I lay there watching the blood flow through the dialyzer and listening to the pulse of the machine for three and a half hours.

The nurse had clicked on the TV, and I remember the Clinton-Monica Lewinsky fiasco interrupted the soap operas. Although I tried to stay awake to see what the hullabaloo was about, eventually I drifted off to sleep, only to be awakened later by the dull beeping of the dialyzer signaling that my first treatment was over.

Dialysis didn't hurt. Since I received it through a catheter, I didn't have to encounter any needles gouging into my vein. I don't know what I expected, but I remember the exhaustion, the slight dizziness, and a sudden need to rest my head on the arm of the dialysis chair. But I fought the urge because I didn't want to succumb to the fatigue. I had to stay strong and continue to tell myself I was not sick. Thus, instead of using the wheelchair near my bed, I was determined to walk back to my room.

Almost immediately after the machine stopped, the nurse walked into the room, clicked off the machine, masked herself and me, disconnected the tubes, and closed off the catheter.

Dialysis healthcare providers do not like catheters because of their potential to cause infection. Some patients with catheters have experienced severe infection, which settled in the lungs, the back, and other areas of the body. Consequently, those receiving dialysis are encouraged to be extremely careful in their physical activities and other lifestyle habits. Intense exercising, extended showering, and anything else that might get the catheter wet are highly discouraged because of the possibility of infection. One hemodialysis patient ended up in a wheel chair from an infection; another got an infection in his back, which resulted in his permanent use of a walker. Clearly, the catheter is a temporary measure until the patient is able to get a fistula or a graft.

A fistula, the preferred access for dialysis because of its effectiveness and minimal potential for infection, is the joining of a vein to an artery at the wrist to provide a more natural access for dialysis. After the surgery, the patient is expected to exercise the hand in order to develop the fistula into something that looks similar to an acorn beneath the skin. That way, once the dialysis needles (one-eighth inch in diameter) are inserted into the fistula, blood can circulate from the body to the machine and back again.

Since I did not yet have a fistula, the goal was to get one as soon as the procedure could be scheduled. The same physician who placed the first and second catheter also performed this particular surgery. After awakening from the procedure, I noticed the forked scar about an inch long on my wrist, and when I touched it, I felt a throbbing motor-like sensation, which I learned later is called a "thrill". I raised my wrist to my ear and heard a murmur, which was actually the pulsating of the blood. The physician, concerned about the success of the procedure, came to see me several times after the surgery to check to see if the fistula had begun to work. Feeling my wrist and listening for the sound of blood flow, he said on one occasion, "I stayed up most of the night worrying about this. You need this fistula to work!"

As the physician seemed concerned about the procedure, I grew anxious about it as well. I didn't need to have to go through this tedious procedure again. Plus, I knew dialysis worked more effectively through a fistula, and catheters were just a temporary measure.

The catheter was still in my chest and I had to be careful to make sure it didn't slip from the appropriate site. I certainly didn't want to deal with any of infection nor the discomfort of having it replaced, so I tried to make sure the catheter rested securely in position.

*****

One morning before daybreak, while still in the hospital, I awakened to a slippery wetness sticking to my stomach and right side. As I tried to sit up, the sheet stuck to my back as blood gushed from the catheter site and flowed over my stomach and down my side. After clicking on the lights, I noticed blood had soaked into my gown and crusted in places on the sheet. My hospital attire looked as if I had been bludgeoned, and the smell nauseated me.

I rang for the nurse, and after what seemed like an hour of lying in scarlet wetness, a nurse's assistant finally came into the room.

"All right," she said, matter-of-factly. "I see we've got a little blood here. Let's get you cleaned up."

She untied my gown and beckoned me to dump the bloody nightclothes into the hamper and sit in the chair while she changed the bed.

Slightly faint from the blood loss, I sat in the recliner while another assistant began to clean and bandage the access site. When she finished, I leaned back listlessly and propped my head against my hand. Another nurse entered and helped me as I moved unsteadily to the bed, where I waited for the morning light.

Because of the bleeding episode, I had to stay in the hospital a few more days to make sure the catheter site was okay, and that the fistula was still efficiently pumping through my wrist. During the next several days, there were intermittent blood tests and x-rays, and I learned what it is really like being in the hospital for more than a day or two.

There is no personal privacy in a hospital. If your gown happens to open inadvertently, exposing your naked rear end, there is no point trying to pull the material together to cover yourself, even if you are able to do so. If you haven't the physical capability, don't expect the assistants to close the gown for you, unless you ask them.

Another common experience of hospitalization is often the patient's sense of losing control. God help you if you can't help yourself because you are at the mercy of the healthcare providers—the nurses' assistants, the phlebotomists, the doctors, the dieticians—everybody, excluding yourself, has some control over your life. I always found it interesting how some of the hospital staff, especially the nurses, spoke to me as if I were a child, or an old woman with hearing problems. Moreover, they almost always spoke in first person plural. I assume they meant well, but I hated the lack of personhood attached to the reference.

"Well, good morning. How are *we* today? Did *we* eat all of our breakfast? Did *we* make a pee pee today?

Sometimes employees who felt comfortable with me after a period of time and assumed I wouldn't report them, complained about their supervisor's attitude, the work schedules, or even a co-worker's negligence, almost as if I were a union representative. I smiled politely and whispered, "Oh, my goodness," or "That's not good," or something equally non-committal, but tried to show concern about their plight, in spite of my fatigue and weariness. Such a response was generally sufficient, as noted in one woman's smile and pat on my blanketed leg as she exited the room.

Hospital employees are certainly interesting people, but no more so than the bureaucracy. For example, the regiment of aftercare for my thyroidectomy, and the ten-day low-iodine diet following the last of the Cytomel pills, was quite an adventure. I started the diet on or about the same day as I began my dialysis. A few days after beginning the diet in the hospital, I had to take three tablets that were unavailable in the admitting hospital. Therefore, I had to be transported by ambulance on a stretcher to another hospital just to take these three pills. I couldn't understand why someone from the neighboring hospital couldn't have delivered the medicine or sent it by messenger. Why did I have to travel from one hospital to another just to take three pills?

Perhaps the change in venue had something to do with radioactivity since I was headed for a nuclear medicine department.

Though I complained about the bureaucracy involved in such a decision, the trip was an interesting change from the usual hospital routines. The drivers, two black men about twenty-something, reminded me of some of the guys I went to high school with in North Carolina. One was a kind of "down home" young man, who loved to talk about his accomplishments and goals, and seemed to be delighted I was interested in his conversation. As I lay on the stretcher listening to the zooming of the ambulance and the driver's chatter, I thought about how we meet and interact with people, if only for a little while, and learn something about their dreams. People seem to enjoy talking about their dreams, probably because it makes the dreams seem real.

This young man, the driver, enjoyed movies and music, and said he was a songwriter. His uncle had written the oldie, "Can I Have a Talk with You?" This song established a kind of connection between us because I knew and loved the lyrics and the tune. We sang some of the song together, as he smiled and flirted. I enjoyed the playacting because for a few minutes, I was no longer in the ambulance on my way to a hospital. I was in high school—a senior, planning for college. My boyfriend was going to another college, but we would be near each other.

> Can I have a talk with you?
>
> Can I make your dreams come true?
>
> Can I? Can I? Can I?[1]

The other young man—big, stocky and sullen, sat in the passenger's seat and remained quiet during our song. He frowned and appeared to sulk much of the time. In fact, he seemed to carry anger in the tilt of his head and the crook of his neck. There was, however, one thing the two of them had in common—their discontent with their working situation. The talkative one made the comments, while the sullen one grunted or said, "Yeah," under his breath. They looked forward to the weekends, the talkative one said, because "Then we work every blue moon." They complained about the dispatcher, and the talkative one said he hoped she didn't make it through the night.

God! What does that mean? "Is she sick?" I asked, raising my head slightly from the stretcher.

"Nope, not that I know of." The talkative one kept driving, while the other one laughed under his breath.

"Just hope she don't make it through the night," he said again.

"What a terrible thing to say!" I eased back on the stretcher.

"Naw," the talkative one said. "That'll be good for her, believe me."

I think if I had been in the ambulance a little longer, I would

---

[1] Kendricks, Eddie. "Can I." All by Myself. Tamla (Motown), 1971.

have discovered the source of their hatred for this woman, but the drive was too short. Through innuendoes and agitated laughter, I learned that these young men felt the dispatcher made their work lives hell.

I wanted to probe the situation, to tell them to focus on their dreams and forget this woman because one day, they might not even remember her name. Besides, their dreams were worth so much more, but before I realized it, the two were opening the ambulance doors and lifting me on the stretcher to the ground at the nearby hospital. After they wheeled me to the registration desk, I waved a feeble hand and thought about these young men who were worth so much more than they seemed to think. For a brief while, they had taken my mind away from the hospital and dialysis and pills, and given me something else to think about.

In a few minutes, however, white coats, blue uniforms, silver stethoscopes, and pale green walls—all brought me back to the world I had to deal with. To take three pills, I had to register, wait for an assistant to administer the medicine, and linger to see if there would be any reaction. Nothing happened. However, I had to wait for what seemed like hours for an ambulance to take me back to the primary hospital. One of the assistants came to the waiting room and asked me if I knew which ambulance service brought me to the hospital.

"Do I *need* to know?" I asked indignantly. I learned I had come to this hospital because it had the nuclear medicine division. Given this information, one would think the hospitals would have their transportation schedules in order.

"Well?" He threw up his hands and began walking away. "Let me check."

This was a dilemma. I was tired and ready to go back to the hospital where I was an inpatient, but I was imprisoned in this waiting room with no information. The admitting hospital couldn't give us the name of the ambulatory service that had brought me to the nuclear medicine site, and everybody was throwing up their hands in ignorance. As I watched this situation unfold in chaos, I was amazed that anyone with my circumstances ever left the hospital with her or his mental faculties intact. Nothing is more indicative of patients' need to be in charge of their own healthcare than being in a hospital.

Another such hardship for me was adhering to the low to non-iodine diet, designed to rid my body of the element and prepare it for a scan. Between two of the many surgeries, I began the diet at home, and with the help of my husband, completed the appropriate shopping and progressed into the routine. It was torturous. I rarely cook with salt or use it on my food; yet, cooking without salt is nothing like eliminating all the iodine from your diet. This meant using only distilled water for drinking, eliminating iodized salt and food with salt, and cooking almost everything. Prepared foods were out of the question. As for distilled water, there is really no way to describe it other than to say the only similarity between distilled water and regular water is its wetness. Any salt had to be non-iodized, the bread made of non-iodated dough, and condiments were almost non-existent. I could have none of the usual goodies such as cheese, regular bread, or crackers, and I couldn't eat in any restaurants. Everything was as bland as a Communion wafer.

I thought I would gain weight during the time I was on the diet, since I was no longer taking the Cytomel (thyroid medicine), but instead I lost weight. Before the diet was over, I had gotten to the point where I could barely stand the sight of food and ate almost nothing. I can't imagine a food regimen worse than a non-iodine diet.

There was some confusion about the diet in the hospital. Possibly because there was too much going on with me and there were too many doctors involved, a problem of coordination of information emerged. My primary care physician, the ear, nose and throat specialist, the nephrologist, the endocrinologist and the vascular surgeon were all involved in my healthcare. The endocrinologist, who did not even know the vascular surgeon, had readmitted me to the hospital and prescribed the non iodine diet, information only I seemed to know. When the food service brought my lunch, the menu consisted of everything I was not supposed to eat—turkey sandwich with mayo and regular bread, tomato soup, and canned fruit cocktail. When the kitchen staff served the lunch and I mentioned the non-iodine diet, they acted as if they knew nothing about it. After I sent the food back, a nurse came in asking about the diet. "What is that?" She asked with an attitude of annoyance.

I tried to explain. "My endocrinologist prescribed it because I …"

"Well, sweetheart, I didn't see anything like that in your chart. We'll just have to contact your doctor." Shaking her head and sighing, she mumbled something as she left the room.

Three mealtimes passed before the staff was able to straighten out my food requirement. Every once in a while, I had my daughter sneak in some fresh unsalted nuts, which she had dry-roasted at home. These nuts actually helped to control the nausea brought on by the entire regimen. Nevertheless, I had to finish the diet in order to undergo the thyroid scan and the subsequent ingestion of radioactive iodine.

*****

The night before the morning of the scan, I lay awake listening to a patient intermittently calling for his mother and people he referred to as Harry and Elizabeth. He howled all night, but nobody seemed to pay him any attention. When a nurse came into my room to check my vitals, I asked about the noisy man down the hall, and she said he was one of the patients from the nursing home who hollers all the time. "We're used to it now," she said, pulling the blanket up to my neck. "He never has any visitors, but he'll be all right."

After the nurse left, I lay there thinking about old people.

DUCK SUMMER: *MY ODYSSEY AS A DIALYSIS PATIENT*

What must it be like to be old, sick, disoriented, alone, and trying to recapture a world that is long gone? Perhaps in their mind, they are as young as they ever were, but the body and circumstances are not willing to cooperate. I imagined the old man lying shriveled like a late autumn leaf, barely breathing, but envisioning himself a young man again with Harry and Elizabeth. I couldn't help but feel a sense of loss for the man who yelled all night because I believed he was trying, subconsciously, to get back to a happier time and place, one of youth and joy. By pre-dawn, he became silent and I imagined he had found Harry and Elizabeth.

After a while, just as a slight hint of pink in the eastern sky began to challenge the darkness, another nurse came into the room and told me that I needed to bathe and prepare to go somewhere.

"Where?"

"I don't know. It wasn't on the chart. All it said was that you were supposed to go somewhere. Round here people just have to go to different places. Don't you know?" She snatched the blanket away from my chest.

Of course, I knew where I was going, but it would have been more reassuring if the nurse had known as well. I was bothered because she was my nurse for the morning and she didn't demonstrate enough initiative or concern to give me, her patient, any significant information. "Good thing I can talk," I said coolly.

The nurse shrugged and grinned as if I had caught her stealing. "They'll be here for you in a few," she said, leaving the room. "Be ready, now," echoed faintly from the corridor.

In less than a half hour, I was on my way back to the nuclear medicine facility at the hospital where I had gone to take the pills. The same two young men brought in the stretcher and had me on my way. I had come to the end of my non-iodine diet and I had to have a body scan to make sure there were no abnormal cells present.

In a cold windowless room, a technician instructed me to lie on what looked like a "cooling board." I climbed to the sheet-covered table and lay flat on my back. Looking up at a big metal case so close to my face, I could smell the breath of the person who preceded me and practically taste the metal trim. The technician told me to lie very still, keep my shoulders flat to the board, and look directly above me. I thought I could manage okay, until I learned I had to remain motionless for more than an hour and a half.

When the scan was complete and I tried to get up, my body clung to the board like metal to a magnet. I struggled again and this time the technician raised her hand to help me off the table. From the scanning room, she sent me to another room, where a much younger technician, who "up-talked" in a whiney voice, ordered me to lie on another table for forty minutes. Unlike the technician before, who tried to answer some of my questions, this technician knew nothing, and responded as if her words had been recorded. "I just do the scan. You'll have to speak to your doctor."

After I completed this testing, the technician pointed me towards still another room where I sat in a chair for more x-rays. This time, she told me the radiologist would read the pictures and talk to the staff doctor, the staff doctor would talk to my doctor, and my doctor would eventually let me know something. I hated the amount of time hospitals take to get life and death information to the patient. With such serious testing, why couldn't I get the results with the same determination and expediency with which they checked on my insurance?

When I returned to the primary hospital, each day seemed longer than the last. Reading put me to sleep. Watching television was boring, and I seemed to have lost whatever hopeful outlook I might have had.

DUCK SUMMER: *MY ODYSSEY AS A DIALYSIS PATIENT*

A couple of days after the scan, as I tried again to watch television, I heard that some guy named McGuire had surpassed Roger Maris's home run record. A Cincinnati news crew did a roaming interview about the historical accomplishment. When the reporter asked one woman what she thought of the home run record, she replied, "Oh my God! Oh my God! He should run for President!" She shouted, looking at the camera as if she were trying to see herself.

"What!" I found myself laughing. "Unbelievable."

It was not very long, however, that TV news turned from McGuire to the impeachment of President Clinton. His alleged involvement with Monica Lewinsky and the girl's "friend," Linda Tripp, were all over the television. I watched the debacle and enjoyed the different responses from some of the hospital staff when they caught a glimpse of the television. Everyone who entered the room had a comment; in fact, some were so passionate about the story, they obviously forgot why they came into my room.

I soon clicked off the T. V. and turned onto my side away from it. I didn't want to hear any more discussion about McGuire, Clinton, Monica Lewinsky or any of the other "TV people," whose lives were far removed from my own, especially now. Whether McGuire was the greatest athlete or not, whether Clinton was lecherous or not, or whether he would or wouldn't be impeached, did not change the fact that my kidneys had failed, and I had to do dialysis again two days from now.

Listlessly, I lay looking towards the window at the white sun slicing through the room and cutting across the bed. I realized that deep inside I was angry. Why was I here? Why was this happening to me? Why were all the people focused on the White House scandal, a baseball triumph, when this hospital and others were filled with people clinging to their lives or wasting away waiting for tests and diagnoses? Then, what about all the people who would eventually confront life-altering health crises? Like me, for example, this dialysis *thing* was surely going to cause drastic changes in my life. I was angry, very angry, but a bigger problem was that there was no object to my anger.

So I turned on myself. When the kitchen staff brought me my last few non-iodine meals, I ate as little as possible. Besides being sick of the monotonous food, I began to see dialysis as a long lonely road of pain and exhaustion. I sank into a depression, and all the discordant sounds bounced from the walls to my bed and circled around me. A song I hadn't thought of or heard since I was in high school rambled through my head, and I wondered if all the medicine had affected my brain.

> I can't get no sleep on this noisy street
>
> I got to move, I got to move
>
> I got to find me a quiet place.[2]

In spite of my escalating depression, every now and then there were situations in the hospital that held me slightly above the abyss. For example, the first time I shared a room during this hospital stay came on the same day I had been warring with depression. The staff moved into the room a friendly Fundamentalist middle-aged white woman who talked incessantly about her church, the new young pastor the church had recruited from Kansas, and how she looked forward to his visiting her in the hospital. Filled with information on how her church fought racism, she talked about some of the oldest members who had marched with King when they were younger, and how some of the youth were engaged in multiculturalism. She said she was extremely pleased with the "racial progress of her community" and that her mission was to recruit some of "the urban population" to attend. She beamed with pride.

---

[2] Mimms, Garnet & The Enchanters. "A Quiet Place." Cry Baby. United Artists, 1964.

Shortly before the evening meal, a young Black male nursing assistant entered and asked her if she were ready for her bath.

"Anytime." She looked up at him and smiled.

"You want to do it or do you want me to do it?" He tilted his head slightly, waiting for her to respond.

My roommate glared up at him with her mouth hanging open far enough to push the chart the young man held into it. For a couple of minutes, she didn't respond, but lay staring like a woman facing the electric chair. "No, No, I can do it!" She swallowed, but clearly tried to conceal her shock. Her face turned as red as a pepper.

The young man hunched his shoulders. "It's up to you."

I turned my head away, laughing silently and thinking, she nearly went into a coma at the thought of a twenty-something man, Black at that, asking her if she wanted him to bathe her.

When he was probably far down the hospital corridor, she took a deep breath and slowly eased back on the bed, shielding herself and her pride with the sheet and blanket.

She was still lying protectively beneath the linen when a nurse entered informing me I would be discharged the next morning.

Chapter 7

A NUCLEAR EXPLOSION

Monday morning, September 14, I had to return to the Hosptial with the nuclear medicine unit to receive radioactive iodine at 10:30. Since I was also scheduled for dialysis that morning, it just made sense to dialyze there as well.

When I arrived at the hospital around 5:15, several people lingered outside the Hemodialysis unit waiting to go in, but the automatic doors weren't working. Those in wheel chairs generally showed no expression, as if this were just a typical morning. A few slept on gurneys with their hands folded across their stomachs, or along their sides, while fluid dripped into the IV. Others leaned against the smudged green wall, apparently not caring if the doors opened or not. As for me, I wanted to twitch my nose like the character on the old television series, "Bewitched," and make the whole scene vanish.

The waiting outside the dialysis unit was exacerbated by my fatigue. The non-iodine diet had all but destroyed my appetite, and since I had not eaten a full meal in almost three weeks, I was exhausted. But at least I could walk into the waiting room, while most of the other patients wrestled with either wheelchairs or gurneys. One woman, white, who looked to be about fifty-something, had lost both legs just below the knees, and also had a hole in her neck out of which dangled a white tube, probably for speaking. She had lost one or two fingers recently, since they appeared freshly bandaged. There were others who had suffered the damages of heart disease, diabetes, strokes, cancer, and a range of other debilitating illnesses. The waiting room for dialysis looked like a war zone with battle-scarred victims scattered throughout the area.

Eventually with a jangling of keys, two security guards, clearly unmoved by the scene, arrived and began to work on the doors. At first, nothing happened, but after a while the doors sprang open and the wheelchairs and gurneys rolled into the dialysis unit like freight train boxcars.

I had a problem getting dialysis that morning. A kink had developed in the port over the weekend, and although I phoned the doctor-on-call for my regular vascular surgeon, no one ever returned the call. On Monday morning, therefore, the doctor in the dialysis unit had to remove the kinked port and replace it with a straight one. With a little numbing medicine, the procedure began.

The doctor pulled a bloody plastic tube from my chest and neck and inserted another one. As he inserted the new tube, I could feel it sticking in my neck from the inside and then clawing around for the right place in my chest. Finally, the doctor assumed the tube had dropped in the right place and called for a chest x-ray. The x-ray showed that the "wire" was, in fact, accurately placed, but the technicians had to cut the dialysis time short because I needed to be in Nuclear Medicine by 10:30 AM.

In Nuclear Medicine, I waited about twenty minutes before a young woman from the scanning room beckoned me to follow her down the hall. She poured into what looked like a half thimble, a brown metallic-looking liquid, the radioactive iodine required as post-operative care for the thyroidectomy. She told me to drink the liquid with a straw and afterwards, pour in water and drink that as well. I stared into the miniature glass, gazing at the tea-like liquid, wondering if it would make my insides glow like a neon sign. But, I was not afraid to drink it because I wanted to do whatever it would take to complete the thyroid therapy. I desperately needed to be finished with this phase of my healthcare.

As soon as I swallowed the tasteless radioactive concoction, I felt woozy.

Rapidly becoming disoriented, I wobbled a few feet down the

hall to a technician. "Should I feel dizzy?" I asked, trying to bring her face into focus.

"Well," she spoke curtly. "Nobody has ever described that to us."

I began to experience a kind of explosion inside my body. A powerful heat began at the top of my head and slowly intensified as it traveled throughout my body. From my head, down my arms, and throughout my chest, the heat swelled in my stomach and fizzled as it reached my groin and legs. The bursts of explosive heat were coming like contractions, first at a slow rate and then gradually more rapidly. In fact, they started to come at a pace where all I could do was catch my breath and prepare for the next one. I thought if I could just get outside the hospital, and breathe non-medicinal air, I would feel better.

By the time I reached the valet area, however, the explosions were coming at the rate of about one a minute, and I had begun to vomit. I fell against a pillar at the entrance of the hospital and threw up again in the midst of another internal explosion. I leaned there heaving and spitting up liquid for what seemed like an hour. A few people passed by, and I could see their mouths moving, but I couldn't hear them because a ringing had begun in my ears. The sounds around me seemed to be coming from very far away. Finally, a young black woman dressed in hospital green came by and I reached to her.

"Help me . . . help me, please," I heard myself saying in a voice that sounded as if it were coming from a barrel of water. "Would you please get someone from Nuclear Medicine? I'm sick." I couldn't stand erect, so I remained bent at the middle, clutching my stomach and heaving when I was not vomiting.

The young woman left to get help and returned quickly. "What is your name?"

"Angelene," I struggled to say.

"Ms. Angelene, do you go to church?"

"Yes," I said and heaved again.

"Well, would you mind if I prayed?" She held my hand.

By then, I was thankful someone was praying for me, because I believed I was dying. I felt her comforting hand on my back, but her voice had begun to fade.

A short while later, I heard the echo of someone's yelling, "They haven't come for her yet! What the hell is Nuclear Medicine doing? Why was she out here alone? This is crazy!"

"Take her to emergency," someone shouted among a group of people in green and white coming towards me. Soon two people helped me to a wheelchair and wheeled me back into the hospital.

"It wasn't nothing we gave her," a man's panicked yell came from a desk down the hallway. "Wasn't nothing we gave her. Can't blame us for this."

As I listened to the voices buzzing around me, somebody handed me a telephone. In the midst of a voice from Nuclear Medicine constantly yelling, "Wasn't nothing we gave her," my internist, who had called the hospital, told me it was probably a reaction to the medicine. To be on the safe side, though, she wanted me to be checked out in the emergency room.

By now, the continuing explosions were accompanied by a shortness of breath. One of the attendants pushed me into a small white room and left me. Alone again, I felt the walls begin to close in on me, and I finally managed to raise my weakened voice to the emptiness around me. "Isn't anyone going to help me?"

A technician came to the door, but he didn't enter. "Just a minute, Miss. We have to test what you threw up in order to make sure you didn't contaminate yourself."

Even in my desperation, the technician's comment made no

sense. So I was contaminating myself with my own medicine?

The explosions were still erupting throughout my body. I tried to bend from the waist and grasp my knees to shield myself from the inferno in my stomach, but the ringing in my ears became maddening. Leaning there with my head almost in my lap, I figured I must be in hell, and that I would remain there until I completely burned from the inside out. What was happening to me? Why wouldn't anyone help me?

After a while, a woman came near me with some kind of hand-held machine that I took to be a radiation detector. Slowly waving it around me, she stood close to the door, distancing herself from me as if my flesh exuded poisonous gas. When she was satisfied I wasn't contaminated, she wheeled me to the emergency room. All this time, I was too weak to hold up my head and it bobbed drunkenly over my lap. By the time I reached the emergency room, I could barely raise it.

"Sign here," a clerk said, pointing to an insurance form. "And if you can't, Dear, just put an X."

The sounds were distorted and I could hardly understand. I thought my life was oozing from my body. I tried to sit up, but the most I could manage was to lean my head on the clerk's desk. I closed my eyes and prayed for some relief from the fire that rolled through my body. If I were dying, then I hoped that God would be merciful and take me into His kingdom, a kingdom that had to have cooling waters, sweet fresh air, and a place I could rest.

The fire had burned out all my energy by the time a nurse came and wheeled me into a section of the emergency room where nurses and technicians scurried about like drunken bees. Lying flat on my back and trying to catch my breath, I heard someone say something about an allergic reaction to the radioactive iodine. I also think I heard that I needed a shot. Anyway, after feeling the pricks of two shots, the heat explosions ceased immediately, my pulse slowed, and I stopped digging my nails into my palms.

I took a deep breath as I heard my husband's voice over my head. He was lifting my hand to his chest, but I could tell from the lines in his forehead and his twisted smile, he was angry and afraid, and wasn't sure where to direct the anger. The only name he knew was my primary physician, the least of the offenders; thus, he attacked her as an inefficient coordinator of my case. I defended her until I was exhausted, pleaded with him not to call her and complain. She was really helping me.

God showed up. He probably was there all along, but He wanted to see if any of these people were doing their jobs. I rebounded quickly after the shots, and I wanted to go home. The emergency room doctor assured my husband I was okay, but my husband didn't think I should leave the hospital. He couldn't easily forget the vision of my lying on the stretcher with only the whites of my eyes showing when he came into the emergency room. Because he had to return to work and would have to leave me alone, he preferred my staying in the hospital where I would have around-the-clock attention. Although that made sense, I was insistent I was not staying in the hospital another minute.

I left that afternoon, but I had to return a few days later for a scan. The doctor wanted to make sure I had not lost the radioactive iodine when I became ill. I guess I didn't, since I didn't hear anything about it in the scan report.

I did learn, however, that I probably became ill because I had too many things scheduled in one day. Dialysis and radioactive iodine therapy in a single morning might just be too much for the system, especially when the system is already vulnerable.

Shouldn't I have been informed?

Chapter 8

A JOURNEY OF ONE'S OWN

For all of its promise as a miraculous life-sustaining treatment, dialysis can be a tough journey, often fraught with depression, loneliness, and fear.

I learned quickly after I had been diagnosed with renal disease that I couldn't depend on the medical system to teach me the complexities of my illness. Nobody was going to educate me about kidneys and the details of how they function or what happens when they cease to work. I was not a medical student; I was a patient, struggling in a world I thought I knew, when in reality, I knew very little. While I put on a confident and stern face, I was really afraid.

My fear of what I didn't know added to my loneliness. Fairly soon during the downward course to renal failure, it was clear this experience was not going to be one the ad agencies might want to use in the hospital's brochures. I was not the only patient and the doctors did not have an infinite amount of office time to give me all the details of my disease. Nurses weren't going to run to my bedside each time I coughed, nor were they going to spend all of their time trying to figure out how to help me. I was in the real world, where HMO's, PPO's and other Machiavellian insurance plans too often dictated doctor-patient contact.

Between the demands of telephones and pagers, physicians were short on reassuring conversations. Social workers, clutching notes on the patient's medications, don't know what to say to bring comfort, and technicians are trained to do their job, not to talk. As hospital personnel shuffle the patient from medical offices to registration stations to labs, none of them provide details about the scheduled services or show much concern about the patient's well-being. Nobody seemed to know anything and if they did, they weren't talking. Sometimes I felt as if I were a condition to be dealt with, an ailment sitting alone watching and worrying.

Dialysis would be less intimidating if patients were informed more thoroughly in the beginning about what to expect. One of the women I met after I began treatment told me she was admitted to the hospital before anyone mentioned to her anything about a procedure. "You have renal failure," her doctor told her as she lay in the hospital bed.

"How long do I have?" She asked, thinking she must be terminal.

Although the woman was diabetic, her doctor had not given her any information about kidney failure as part of the diabetes discussion. Or, if he did, she obviously didn't understand or retain it. The point is that most patients approaching dialysis have little, if any, information about it. Even those who know of its inevitability in their lives and engage in significant reading don't have enough information.

I had known for years that I might have to go on dialysis some day, and although I didn't allow myself to believe it until my kidneys began to show significant decline, I nevertheless read about renal failure, dialysis treatment, kidney transplant, and anything I could find related to kidneys. Moreover, I talked to people who were on dialysis and those who had undergone transplants, and I read the Kidney Newsletter. While I was more knowledgeable than many patients, I had no idea how much I still did not know.

The orientation I attended before I began the dialysis process was not very helpful. Along with two other women, who appeared to be relatives or friends, I listened to two presentations—one by a relatively well-informed nurse and the other by a part-time social worker. The nurse discussed the various types of dialysis, food and fluid restrictions, and answered a few questions. Apparently compassionate and knowledgeable, she also talked about the function of the kidneys and how the artificial kidney would resume the work of the failed organs. With a noticeable slant towards peritoneal dialysis (dialysis performed through a tube surgically inserted in the stomach, where exchanges of fluid are performed daily), the nurse showed a video, emphasizing it and illustrating young and old talking about how easy life was while undergoing this form of dialysis. The video was essentially a commercial for peritoneal dialysis.

The social worker, on the other hand, focused primarily on insurance issues. Like a student with a boring assignment, she explained a few things about Medicare, barely answered our questions, and rushed through her presentation. I assumed she must have been poorly paid and/or had little or no interest in her job, since she appeared to be anxious to get through the material.

Near the end of the session, the nurse asked what we thought about the prospect of going on dialysis, given what we had heard. One woman, fiftyish, gazed at the table as if she had gotten lost in it. Then taking a deep breath, she rested face in her hands and mumbled, "I'd rather be dead."

Nobody said a word.

There was no sharing. None of us were willing to open up about anything. Instead, we sat at the table as if our common illness were contagious; in fact, we didn't even make eye contact.

The other woman, who had obviously already begun dialysis, tried to console the despondent one. "I felt the same way when I started," she said. "I didn't know anything then, but now I'm glad I did it." In a wheelchair and using oxygen, she appeared to be suffering from some other illnesses. As I glanced from one to the other, I wondered what had hastened their renal failure. Was it diabetes, high blood pressure, a virus, or did it just happen? What had their journeys been like?

But what brought them here was perhaps less important than

what now lay ahead. The brief orientation prepared us for nothing. We needed at least a two-day symposium with doctors, nurses, technicians, and maybe even a few patients, who could speak to the specific aspects of the process. This kind of program would have given us more information on the procedure, what it is and what it does, the people involved in it, the necessary medications and their purposes, the possible complications, diet and fluid restrictions, and the differences among hospital facilities, off-site clinics and home dialysis.

Most people outside this dialysis world know almost nothing about the procedure, or the toll it often takes on the patient's well-being. I found it interesting, yet isolating and depressing, the way some people responded when they learned I was on dialysis.

"What's that?"

I always tried to explain the procedure simply. "Well, there's a machine that filters the blood taken from your body. The blood circulates through a tube with a large needle usually stuck into the arm and blah, blah, blah.

"Oh my God! How awful! Does it hurt? How long do you have to do it?"

Those who knew that dialysis was somehow connected with kidney failure glibly told me that I could "just get a kidney," as if it were sold from a vending machine.

Even those with some familiarity could not comprehend how I could have renal failure, given I didn't have high blood pressure or diabetes, two primary factors in kidney disease. A "mere" chronic inflammation just didn't make sense to them.

Also, the people close to me didn't seem to understand my renal failure and certainly didn't know how dialysis worked. In their lack of awareness, they didn't know what to say. For example, instead of my mother's asking questions about the status of my kidneys before they completely failed, she said in her endearing way, "Lord Jesus, I pray you won't have to go on that machine. I heard about it."

When I became ill and ended up on "the machine," she repeated each day I underwent dialysis, "You had to go on that machine today, didn't you? Umph! Umph! Umph!"

Although she lived in another part of the country, I could see her shaking her head with each word, and I knew that was her way of saying, I'd trade places with you in a minute if it would spare you that machine.

Church members and friends didn't seem to want to know about the dialysis process, but instead commented on how tough I was and how good God is. "Girl, the Lord is able, and you know you can handle this."

People at the University had heard I was ill during much of the summer. One of my friends told me some of my colleagues were questioning her. When I inquired about the gossip, she shook her head and said, "It's just too terrible to repeat." Such a response sent my imagination spiraling. Since very few people knew the specifics of my health problems, I had obviously fallen victim to the speculation mill: Maybe I was struggling with something terminal. Perhaps I was on chemotherapy. Or maybe I was suffering from something unmentionable. Tongues probably flapped like a loose screen door in a storm.

During one of those times when I was released from the hospital and went to campus, some of my colleagues looked at me as if I had come back from the dead.

However, when they learned I had renal failure and had begun dialysis, the idle speculation and gossip turned into their attempt at words of assurance.

"Girl! You a tough sister. You can deal with this. Sisters pretty much deal with anything. We got to, girl! And I don't know anybody that can handle this any better than you."

I hated these remarks. All they did was prohibit me from admitting I had the same strengths and weaknesses as any other human being. My friends' comments were tied to the concept of Black women as superhuman, capable of enduring the most dreadful situations stoically. Although they knew little about dialysis, they assumed whatever it was and however it worked, I could handle it. I was a *real* Black woman.

I resented the assumption I could handle dialysis with ease. I grew angrier at each presumption about my strength, and how I was such a good role model for people with chronic health issues. They didn't leave space in their minds for me to be vulnerable, lonely, scared, and sometimes depressed. Even more troubling, I'd begun to feel I had to live up to these expectations. In many ways, I allowed others to shape my response to my own health problems.

Few could tell I had any health problems from looking at me. I hid my disfigured arms under sleeves and shielded the swollen veins in my neck behind collars, despite the weather. I never mentioned dialysis and never ever complained. Even when I desperately wanted a soft drink or a tall glass of water to moisten the dusty coating inside my mouth, I said nothing and instead chewed gum. During the early days, when I still had the catheter in my chest and it itched like a chigger bite, I didn't speak of it. When depression weighed on me like cement, I continued to function as if nothing had changed. I wanted to be what others said I was—the strong Black woman.

There came a time, however, when my resolve to endure weakened. I remember once when I had been in the hospital over a week and things were not going well. (Dialysis patients are known for their stays in the hospital for clotted catheters and fistulas, blood pressure problems, heart malfunctions, etc.). I received word that a woman about three years my junior, had died suddenly. I had been depressed for days, and all I needed was information about the death of a church member and friend to remind me of my own mortality. The news arrived, shocking me out of my role as the strong Black woman. My husband and a few others stood near the bed as I began to weep, the tears gushing from my eyes and streaming down my cheeks. "Am I going to die?" I tried to whisper to my husband through sobs. "Am I going to die, too?"

The question seemed natural to me, especially given the challenges I had been facing for months. Yet, the friend standing on the opposite side of the bed from my husband patted my hand patronizingly and with a look of betrayal, said, "Now, now, I think you just feeling a little sorry for yourself. That's all this is." It didn't seem to occur to her that she was on her feet, while I was lying flat on a hospital bed. Even in my weakness, I became furious. "I'm not entitled?" I turned to the window, my arm resting in the puddle of blood that had seeped from the catheter onto the bed.

I know now that what my friend objected to was the fear she saw in my eyes and heard in my voice. Signs of weakness. As long as I was a tough trash-talking sister, who could deal with almost any problem, she didn't have to adjust to any uncomfortable changes, or confront her own weaknesses and vulnerabilities.

I *did* have a serious health problem and pretending it didn't exist might make her comfortable, but it only depressed me. I was not on dialysis because I wanted to see what it was like: I was on dialysis because I had kidney failure. My kidneys—major organs in my body, were no longer functioning. Other than occupying space, they did nothing. Without an artificial means of replacing their function, I would die. These were the facts, and when I cried or showed fear, my friends were forced to confront the possibility that they too could one day face such an illness.

I didn't want to look into the eyes of others and see their fear either, so I tried to pretend nothing had changed; yet, everything had changed. Dialysis changed the self-controlled woman with a solid grip on the ways of the world into a scared child wading through water with sand bags tied to her legs.

*****

I spent the first six months of my treatment accompanied by fear and loneliness. On Mondays, Wednesdays, and Fridays, from 1:30 to 4:00 in the afternoon, I underwent dialysis. As the afternoon hours are the least favored block of time, newcomers are left with those appointments.

In the early stages of my dialysis, I could not understand why the unit was almost always running behind schedule. It was not long, though, before I had to suck up my self-pity and recognize others whose pain and suffering were greater than my own. Even with barely functioning kidneys, I was in fairly good condition compared to some of the in-patients who were being treated. Moreover, some of the incapacitated patients from nursing homes and other hospitals, with difficulties such as uncontrollable bleeding, dangerously low blood pressure, shortness of breath and sometimes fainting, had to remain in the unit until they recovered. A plethora of other health issues could send the staff into a flurry of life-saving precautions causing a delay in the admission of patients waiting in the dialysis lobby.

After I began to comprehend the nature of the hospital dialysis unit, I appreciated the massive difficulties some dialysis patients could experience, and of course, I then interpreted my own complaining as whining. Furthermore, the situation itself taught me that no amount of fuming, pounding the buzzer, complaining or cursing from patients waiting in the lobby, would take the staff's attention from patients experiencing health crises.

I learned to respect the dedication and professionalism of many of the hospital dialysis personnel because they held the healthcare needs of the patient as the highest priority. In the hospital unit, doctors frequently visited the patients, nurses were highly skilled, and even the technicians appeared devoted to patient health and comfort.

Patient comfort is apparently a significant part of the protocol in hospital dialysis units. For example, during the cleansing procedure, body temperature is reduced, leaving patients uncomfortably cold, sometimes shivering. In these cases, hospitals provide warm blankets, whereas patients at freestanding clinics must supply their own. Also, hospital units offer six-ounce soft drinks to patients who control their fluid intake, and pay special attention to other personal needs. With in-patient illnesses and the drain of the procedure on the body, patient survival would be at risk without the constant attention of the personnel.

*****

While the hospital can be the best place for both dialysis patients needing special care, and those beginning their treatment, it can also be one of the worst, psychologically. Given its focus on the most severely ill renal patients, hospitals can often be devastating to otherwise healthy patients. For example, during my early tenure at the hospital, my dialysis unit or "pod" held three other patients—two who took their treatments in bed because they were debilitated and the other who was in a wheelchair and on oxygen.

Rarely did I see anyone in this particular area whose renal failure was not accompanied by some other devastating illness. One woman, who took her treatments in bed, had to be lifted and changed as if she were a baby. Woefully thin, she whimpered constantly. From where I sat, I could see only her feet and legs, which were stilled with wooden restraints. Her relentless moans, distant and timeless, made me think she was an elderly woman. However, one day when two of the technicians lifted her from her bed, I saw she was indeed quite young, perhaps somewhere between thirty and thirty-five.

DUCK SUMMER: *MY ODYSSEY AS A DIALYSIS PATIENT*

I sank into a deep depression when I learned the woman was a physician, who had an allergic reaction to some medicine taken during her pregnancy. She became completely paralyzed and would probably remain so. I cried for her. Then I prayed she would miraculously rise from her bed like Lazarus from the grave. If she could be healed, then so could we all.

I found some comfort in my assumption that the woman was not fully conscious, since I never saw her talking to anyone. At least she did not have to lie restrained in her bed aware of her helplessness. Perhaps when she regained consciousness, she would be stronger, alert and ready to take some control of her life. However, when she began to receive visits from her daughter and mother, who often sat with her during her treatments, and with whom she quietly conversed, I knew she was aware of her condition and I became even more depressed. Although most of the time, I could see only the bottom of her feet, she became another symbol of dialysis to me—an alert mind, but a non-functioning body. I sank further into despair.

The women's situation and my grief over it reminded me of what the old folks in my hometown had always encouraged the children to do when we could not understand something. "Read the Bible," their voices echoed to me from the distant past. "It's got the answer to everything." In my efforts to deal with the despondency, I went to the Scriptures and while hooked to the machine, I read more of the Bible than I had at any other time since college.

I had to chuckle when my thoughts went back to my college's requirement that we attend chapel three times a week in assigned seats. Maybe the administration knew what they were talking about after all. We thought it was ridiculous at the time, but what other opportunity did we have to sit quietly and reflect, to take a mental break, or to read the Bible? Perhaps, the chapel requirement instilled in me the importance of personal time, and the virtue of patience, which I especially needed in the dialysis chair.

Dialysis stimulated more philosophical and religious questions than ever before. I viewed my renal failure as a kind of test, and thought I could perhaps find the answers or at least some insight in the Bible. With all the women and men in both the Old and New Testaments who had experienced tests of faith and loyalty, I wanted to look again at how they confronted their challenges. How did Job survive and prosper, given all his ordeals? What about Ruth, Naomi, Esther, and Mary? All favored by God, these Biblical figures had something I was struggling with—faith and assurance.

It was also during this period of self-doubt and uncertainty that I frequently thought about death. I like to think that dialysis never so devastated me that I wanted to die, but I did become interested in questions about life and death. Did dialysis mean I was living on borrowed time? How much flexibility was there in my life now that I had to carve out a specific three hours and a half, three days a week, in an already tight schedule? When I went out of town, if I didn't schedule dialysis, I would more than likely feel the effects of fluid retention and an increase of toxins in my blood. If this experience were to characterize my life, how was I ever going to feel hopeful about the future?

Thoughts of death remained with me. Was the afterlife truly a place of peace and joy, springtime flowers and blue skies? Was the old folks' notion that all we had to do in Heaven was spend the time praising God, true? Was there really no such thing as renal failure in death? Could I get back my life in death?

Warring with inner turmoil and conflicts, I looked up one day to find the hospital chaplain standing near my chair. I had noticed his stopping by the pods to talk to patients, but I hadn't given him any indication I was interested. Hence, the first time he came to my chair, I girded my emotions and donned a detached front. I was in no mood for religious talk, especially not the simple answers and rehearsed platitudes I expected from a chaplain on payroll.

To my amazement, the chaplain, a white man who reminded me of the aging Henry Fonda, didn't talk religion in the way I expected. There were no discussions of Heaven and hell, repentance, God's will, and the like. Instead, he wanted to know who I was and in a subtle way, what was really going on in my head and heart. Before I realized it, I was expressing my ideas about many issues—dialysis, God, my faith, health, and expectations for the future, the physicians, and hospital bureaucracy. His matter-of-fact demeanor made it easy for me to articulate the uncertainties and contradictions in my life.

He helped me to accept that it was okay to have unsettling feelings about God. My family had raised me to think that any unfavorable thoughts about Him would initiate His wrath. None of them ever talked about a God with a sense of humor; however, the Chaplain encouraged me to consider the possibility. If God loved me, truly loved me—a human being, then the same God knew of my frailties and probably found it amusing that I tried so hard not to be angry with Him when He did things I didn't like.

As he and I debated issues of faith and talked about Native American folklore, world religions and other academic topics, he recommended certain texts I should study. Of course, I reciprocated by suggesting certain books by African Americans he needed to read.

With the passing of time, it became apparent that the Chaplain was benefiting as much from our conversations as I was. Eventually I did, in fact, want to talk about God, and I expected a Chaplain, of all people, to have the answers. How did God make choices? Was there some divine plan where everyone was just a robot with no free will? Or, were we the cause of the things that happened to us? Had I, in some way, mistreated my body and instigated my renal failure?

Instead of answering my questions, the Chaplain took the Socratic approach, and asked questions in return, which helped me to focus. After a while, I came to understand that what I wanted desperately was to understand God. I needed also to be sure He had nothing against me personally, that He actually liked me, and was pleased that I had tried to gain His favor.

I remembered the many times my mother had told me there was nothing I could do to gain God's favor. He would love me no matter what because that is who He is. I heard, but I do not think I really understood. How could I relate to God if I were not trying to gain His favor? What could I do? Did I not have to do something? On a journey such as dialysis, I needed answers. The Chaplain didn't have any, but he certainly helped me raise different questions.

When my treatment time changed from mid-afternoon to early morning, I rarely saw him, but I knew he was still coming to the dialysis unit, talking to other patients and trying to help them deal with their situation. He had helped me.

Chapter 9

FISTULAS, CATHETERS, AND GRAFTS

I had a catheter dangling from my chest and a fistula pulsing in my left wrist. The fistula, the connection of a vein to an artery, caused such swelling in my hand from the heavy flow of blood that it looked like a ballooned glove. Eventually, I had to remove my wedding ring because it was strangling the circulation. Soon the surgeon who put the fistula in my arm and the catheters in my chest ordered an ultrasound of my arm. After discovering the fistula was not developing, he scheduled a surgery to prevent the excessive flow of blood to my hand.

After the surgery on the fistula, I began to worry if I would be able to get dialysis through this kind of access. I knew the technicians and the nurses would be using the catheter for a while, but I was also aware that they don't like using catheters as an access for dialysis. Catheters frequently cause blood clots, slow dialysis runs, infections and a plethora of other problems. However, they do not require the development time of grafts and fistulas, and are a temporary measure while dialysis patients wait for the more acceptable access.

My catheters were the accesses from hell. As mentioned earlier, the first one clotted before I ever began dialysis treatments. The second one provided an inefficient dialysis treatment and caused an infection manifesting itself in flu-like symptoms. The objective of any dialysis treatment is to cleanse the blood of toxins, waste, excess fluid and salt that developed since the last treatment. The number of times the blood circulates through the artificial kidney or dialyzer largely determines the effectiveness of the treatment.

Catheters can't sustain a high flow of blood in and out of the body, and often the machine will stop during use. When this happens, the machine begins to beep, signaling a cease in blood flow. When I had my second catheter, from September 4 until December 23, my machine beeped more than an overused microwave. Every time it beeped, it stopped working, and whenever it stopped working, the technician added the time to my dialysis treatment. For example, when my running time was three hours and a half, I might end up at the treatment unit for an additional half hour.

    Blood clots, too, pose a serious threat to good dialysis. One day in December, I stayed in the dialysis unit of the hospital from 1:30 PM, my starting time, until 8:40 PM. The problems started with a clot forming in the catheter. When the technicians tried to flush the catheter as they always do, the saline rushed through the syringe, but produced only a pinkish hint of blood. Sometimes when this happens, especially if there is a small clot, a flush or two of saline will resume the dialysis.

    However, on this particular afternoon, the saline didn't work and the only recourse was urokinase, a substance in limited supply, which takes time to work. Between the times the nurse flushed the catheter with the de-clotting substance and the start of my treatment an hour later, I sat wondering how late it would be before this dialysis experience would be finished.

    I had no idea, however, that before the treatment ended, there would be other problems. Ordinarily I would have been able to leave the dialysis unit three and a half hours after the treatment began. However, within an hour after the catheter started to work, I became seriously ill. With severe chills, a fever of 102.4, and a blood pressure of 223/100, I thought I was dying. The technician and a couple of nurses brought warm blankets to cover me, but with each passing minute my insides seemed to freeze. The uncontrollable shivering and an elevated blood pressure collided in my head and repeatedly exploded. I felt critically ill.

    The chills flabbergasted the nurses and technicians. One of the nurses even said she suspected an infection, but the chills were atypical.

DUCK SUMMER: *MY ODYSSEY AS A DIALYSIS PATIENT*

After giving me some antibiotics, the nurse drew blood for the lab. For a long while, I lay suffering a ghastly headache, which slowly began to subside. When the antibiotic started to take effect, the chills diminished, but my body was sore from the extreme shivering and exhausted from the headache.

When I returned to dialysis for my next treatment, I learned the lab reports showed I had an infection in my blood. As the catheter goes directly into the blood stream, any foreign matter that gets into the blood via the catheter can cause a serious infection. In my case, the infection manifested itself in flu-like symptoms. Infections of a more serious nature, such as infections of the spine, have resulted in either partial or complete paralysis. These conditions are the reasons dialysis nurses and technicians warn patients about the restrictions which govern the use of a catheter.

That morning, the technician didn't hook me to the machine as usual. Instead, a nurse removed the infected catheter and inserted an even more temporary one into my groin for dialysis. After the treatment was over, the nurse removed the catheter, bandaged the area, and told me to watch for any excess bleeding or other signs of infection.

*****

Christmas weekend of 1998, I flew to Delaware to visit my mother-in-law. Having contacted the social worker with a request to schedule my treatment somewhere in the vicinity, I was struggling to maintain some semblance of normalcy. It was not easy. The social worker found a dialysis unit about sixty miles in one direction from my mother-in-law's house, as all of the nearby units were filled to capacity, which is often the case. The drive would take about an hour and a half each way, a total of three hours, and the treatment was another three hours. The time consumption of the on-site dialysis would be about six hours of the three days I planned to spend in Delaware. For this occasion, I decided to forgo my dialysis treatment and called the unit to cancel the appointment. I knew canceling was an unwise thing to do, but I tried to compensate for the negligence by fervently adhering to my diet and fluid restrictions.

Throughout the entire weekend, I craved a diet cola, something on the list of food and drink restrictions because of its high level of phosphorous. Thinking my idea of the good life had been reduced to a soft drink, I could almost taste the sweet cola on my tongue and feel the fizz in my mouth.

With all these difficulties, it is no wonder I began to think dialysis was a death penalty. I had contracted an infection, my catheter only barely worked when it worked at all, and my efforts to go out of town on a holiday was a nightmare. New Castle, Delaware, my destination, was two miles from Wilmington, Delaware and about thirty miles from Philadelphia. With all the hospitals in and around the vicinity of these two cities, I couldn't get a site within sixty miles, which is indicative of the vast number of people with kidney failure.

I had been without an access since my last dialysis treatment. Therefore, when I returned to the hospital for my treatment, one of the nurses summoned a couple of the interns, to take care of the matter. As far as I knew, they were just two people in white coats from somewhere—the sky, for all I knew, but I tried to be calm. From the very beginning of my dialysis treatments, I always tried to be cooperative because I knew that despite the difficulties, inconveniences, and even pain, the healthcare professionals had my best interests in mind. However, had it not been for my assuming I would never have to encounter these two interns again, the experience would have forever tainted my impression of medicine.

The nurse, who remained with me throughout the procedure, ushered me to the gurney and pulled the curtain. Soon the young white woman and young Asian man, both not much older than my daughter of twenty-seven, stood over me, eyeing my neck like it was a good dinner. Pulling her latex gloves on, the woman spoke as if I were deaf. "We want you to hold real still and this won't take long. We're going to put a catheter into your neck."

"My neck! Not my neck!" I rose on my elbows from the gurney. "Can't you put it somewhere else?"

"We have to put it in the neck because there is nowhere else to put it. The groin is much too temporary."

Already I could tell they both had the bedside manner of a gnat.

The nurse grabbed my hand, holding it reassuringly.

I couldn't believe the doctors were going to put this thing in my neck. I had seen patients with the catheter sticking out of the side of their neck like a tusk and I wondered how they could tolerate it. Now here I lay, preparing to have the same thing done to me. Already vanity was creeping into my psyche and I worried about how I would conceal the catheter and try to look normal when I had this *thing* protruding from my neck.

The woman gave me a shot of lidocaine to prepare my neck for the invasion. Awkwardly, she began trying to insert the catheter into the vein, but the pain was so unbearable I retreated in a fetal position.

"This hurts!" I moaned.

She shot me again with more lidocaine and then shoved the catheter in again.

"Just a little while longer and it will be all over," the nurse said.

"But my neck hurts," I reached up to feel it. "And it's already swollen."

"The swelling will go down by tomorrow. It's just lidocaine," the male intern breathed impatiently.

"The swelling is only temporary," the nurse whispered, patting the back of my hand.

The intern pushed the catheter again, but commented that she couldn't seem to get past the scar tissue. Since I had undergone the placement of two other catheters in my chest and surgery on my neck, I was not surprised there was severe scar tissue. The doctor's struggling to get the catheter into the vein was excruciating and I began to feel nauseated. I glanced up to the face of the nurse, who still held my hand, and noticed her eyes were watery. When the intern realized she couldn't get the catheter past the scar tissue, she turned to the Asian intern, who shot me with more lidocaine and started the procedure all over again. He jabbed the catheter into my neck as if he were digging for gold, but he too could not pierce the vein.

Finally, both interns knew they were not going to get this catheter placed, at least not into my neck. By the time they surrendered to the scar tissue, I was nauseated and my neck was so swollen I could see it in my peripheral vision.

"It's the lidocaine," she said. "That's why it's swollen. I told you it would go away overnight."

The interns finally put an access into my groin, but by then I was numb from my neck to my thighs. They could have done most anything and I wouldn't have felt it because the pain they had already inflicted had practically dulled my senses. For the next 36 hours, I vomited, suffered extreme fatigue, and had no appetite. The next time I had a treatment, the nurse who had been with me during the ordeal commented that she didn't know how I lived through the horror. She said I squeezed her hand so tightly she had to use an ice pack on it.

It was more than a week before my neck returned to its normal size. In the interim, I took dialysis through the catheter in my groin, which had to be replaced each treatment to prevent infection. Near the end of the week, which was the day before New Year's Eve, I met with another surgeon who had called me about another neck access. I flat out refused and asked to meet with him at the hospital to discuss the matter.

I had never met the surgeon who was now planning to insert another catheter. This young physician, I discovered, was well established in the field of vascular surgery and had a personality that suggested he had nothing to prove. He appeared to understand my concerns about having a catheter protruding from my neck. Explaining my options, he told me he would put the catheter in the neck, but he would make sure the instrument was not visible. As soon as possible, he noted, I would have to have another access, one that wasn't as susceptible to infection.

On New Year's Eve, I had to be at the hospital by 7:30 for another ultrasound of my arm. The surgeon wanted to see what was happening with my arm. Because the fistula was not developing, I had to undergo a procedure consisting of running a scope up and down my arm for almost an hour. Painless, the ultrasound was more boring than watching the blood flow through the tubes during a dialysis treatment.

After the ultrasound of my arm, I prepared for the surgery scheduled for 11:30 a.m., then rescheduled for 1:00 p.m. due to another patient's emergency. At 12:30, the nurses began the anesthesia in my arm and by 12:45, I was drifting off to that place of absence we go to during surgeries.

I awakened with the catheter in my chest. I felt my neck. There was no swelling and no tubes. After being dismissed into the bright starry New Year's Eve, I decided to attend Watch Night Service at my church.

*****

In January of the New Year, the vascular surgeon who provided the first two catheters decided the fistula was not working and probably never would. In response, he severed the vein from the artery, thus deconstructing the fistula, and put a graft in my lower forearm. By now, I had become a frequent patient at the hospital. Most of the staff in registration, pre-admission testing, and surgery knew me by name. "So, you're back with us again," somebody always announced. "You just can't get enough of us." I still had the third catheter in my chest, but I was happy to have the graft. A six-inch tube under the skin, connecting a vein to an artery, the graft meant that eventually I might not have to worry about infection, blood clots in the tubes, and less than favorable dialysis lab reports.

However, my excitement over the graft was short-lived. Normally it takes about two weeks after the surgeon places the graft in the arm before technicians can use it for dialysis. Before each treatment, one of the nurses puts a stethoscope to the graft to listen for the heightened sound of blood flow. If she hears something like a gushing stream, then the graft is working. When I lifted my arm to my ear, I could also hear the blood roaring through the graft, even without the instrument.

About ten days later, I lay in my bed with my arm against my ear. All I heard was the normal beat of my pulse. No raging waters. No motor rev. I listened again, waiting to hear a functioning graft, but still there was only a slight pulse. I asked my husband to listen for the gushing sound, and he couldn't hear it either. We decided not to panic, but to wait until my next dialysis appointment, when the nurse would check it with her stethoscope.

That Monday, when the dialysis nurse examined my graft, she concluded it had clotted. "Well," she said as if this happens all the time. "You'll have to see the surgeon."

I couldn't believe this was happening again. I was tired of surgeries. Not only was my arm scarred from an automobile accident years earlier, but from the three surgeries on the wrist and the previous one for the graft. My left arm looked as if I had been attacked by a bear. How much more did I have to endure?

My challenges continued the following week when I went back to see the vascular surgeon I had been working with since before the treatments. Although we had not had any success with the fistula or the graft, and we had not achieved optimum effectiveness with the catheters, I still had confidence in him. With his calm and reassuring manner, he had been able to assuage my fear of surgery. He had demonstrated great sensitivity to and concern for my dilemma. Moreover, his mother was a dialysis patient, so I knew he had more than just a professional interest in the problems associated with renal failure.

On the day of my appointment, I waited in one of the examination rooms for what seemed like an hour. Actually, it was more like twenty minutes before he had time to see me. "How are you, young lady?" he asked in the caring tone I had come to associate with him.

"Okay, I guess." I didn't know what else to say, given all the difficulty I had endured for almost five months.

He reached for my hand and stared at the graft. Shaking his head, he gently pressed the stethoscope along the print of the graft.

"I want you to see someone else. He's a surgeon as well, but he is more experienced in these types of procedures than I am. I am a vascular surgeon, as you know. But I don't have as much experience with inserting grafts as he does."

I didn't want to hear this. He was a kind man, a doctor with demonstrated compassion and genuine concern for me as a person with hopes and fears. I didn't want to have to adjust to another surgeon. "No, I don't want to do this. Let's just try it one more time. It'll work. I know it will."

"I think this is best for you. I have tried, but I am not able to do you any good. And I want this to work for you." He hesitated for a few minutes and then continued. "If it were just ego, I would try it again, but it's not ego. You shouldn't have to keep going through this, so I want you to see this other doctor. I have already called him and explained your case."

Tears came. Of all the things I had endured, having to see another surgeon was overwhelming. I composed myself. "I don't want another doctor."

"I'm sorry, but I think he will be able to help you and I haven't been able to." He put the stethoscope on the counter and wrote the doctor's name and number.

"I'll never again get attached to a doctor. Never again." I stepped down from the examination table and reached for my purse. "I'll never get attached again."

The doctor gave me an impassive hug, barely touching my shoulder.

*****

It was over a month before I met with the new doctor. Very different from the previous vascular surgeon, he was abrasive, arrogant, and impatient. He couldn't wait to tell me how fortunate I was to get an appointment with him. "When it comes to grafts," he said. "I am the best." He spent all of ten minutes talking with me about the procedure before he sent me to his assistant to schedule the surgery.

Already, I didn't like him. He seemed to represent the big business of medicine—a corporation for his practice, hundreds of nameless and faceless patients a day farmed out to one intern or another, and an abominable bedside manner. Before I left his office, he and I exchanged a few quick remarks about the procedure as he walked out into the hallway. I sensed he was unaccustomed to patients' asking questions, since another nippy exchange occurred in the hallway of his office when he briskly responded to questions while walking away from me.

Clearly, we didn't endear ourselves to each other.

The surgeon's assistant scheduled the procedure for April, but after all the medical rigmarole, I didn't think I even wanted a graft anymore. The catheter had been performing fairly well, I was getting better chemistry readings, and the flow reached a level of at least 350 on some days. Moreover, with the catheter I didn't have to wait 20 minutes, pressing my arm to stop the bleeding before I could leave the dialysis unit.

There were also other advantages of the catheter. First, unlike with the graft, the technicians didn't have to stick needles a third the diameter of a pencil into the patient's arm for the blood to exit the body through the tube, dialyze, and re-enter through another tube and equally large needle. In fact, after I had been going through dialysis for about nine months, I started to watch people with grafts as they were stuck twice, sometimes four times if they used lidocaine, and I was reminded of how glad I was that I didn't have to endure what must be excruciating pain.

But I needed the graft. I underwent the surgery on April 6, 1999 and awakened from the procedure to a half-moon-shaped nylon tube under the skin of my upper left forearm. Surprisingly, the new surgeon was exceptional in the operating room. Friendly, patient, gentle and meticulous in his every move, he proved he had earned what the old folks used to refer to as "bragging rights." After the surgery, when my husband asked how things went, he said the surgeon looked at him as if to say, "How do you think it went? I'm the best."

I was okay. Smiling at the sound of blood pulsating through my arm, I could feel and hear it through the heavy bandages. What a wonderful sound. I frequently lifted my arm to my ear just to hear "life". The roaring swish was music, singing and sending the sounds throughout my body.

A week and a half later, however, the graft clotted and I was back in the hospital for a de-clotting procedure.

Following the procedure, the graft worked perfectly. When the technician approached the new catheter for use, she asked me if I were planning to use the numbing medicine, lidocaine. "Is that a serious question?" I responded with a tinge of sarcasm. "Of course, I'm going to use the medicine. Why wouldn't I want to dull the pain of that horrendous needle?" I glanced up at the tube with the needle at the end.

The technicians stuck me two times a day, three times a week beginning May 7, 1999, and each time I used lidocaine.

I used lidocaine for approximately two and a half months until I traveled to Richmond, Virginia to attend and participate in a Hurston-Wright Writers' Workshop at Virginia Union University. The workshop lasted a week, which meant I had to take dialysis three times in an unfamiliar location. There, the staff seemed to think using lidocaine was a laughing matter, a joke, and I should be persuaded to take the needles without it.

"Why get stuck four times—two times for lidocaine and two times for the dialysis? Besides, it's better for your graft if you don't use lidocaine."

I had heard that before, but it didn't make any difference. I wasn't even sure I believed it.

Ironically, though, on my first therapy in Richmond, I agreed to try one cite without the lidocaine. I already knew how much the lidocaine needle hurt, although it was about the same size as the needles used to extract blood for lab tests. I figured the dialysis needle would be unbearable. I just couldn't deal with the horrendous pain brought on by such a large needle piercing a tender part of my skin.

The nurses and technicians were persistent. "So you're still going to be stubborn," one of the nurses commented with a gleeful eye. "Up to you, honey. I don't get it, but I guess you do." She prepared my arm for the lidocaine. "Ready, Dearie?"

"Okay, okay." I folded my arm, guarding against the lidocaine needle. "I'm going to try this one time, and then I'll go back to the regular." I unfolded my arm and waited for the nurse to switch needles.

"Up to you, Sweetie." She smiled and winked. "You'll be glad if you do this."

"Ugh," I mumbled. I hated it when the staff called me by those pseudo-endearing names. She needn't think I was afraid of the needle. I just didn't see the sense in the extra pain.

I braced myself for the dialysis needle. Surprisingly, the nurses and technicians were right. Without any lidocaine, the dialysis needle was no more painful than it was with the typical anesthesia. It didn't make much sense to take four needles when two served the need.

I became accustomed to the large needles and discovered a way to avoid most of the pain. Inhaling before the needle pierced the flesh and exhaling as it went through the skin, made the procedure considerably less painful. In fact, from that first experience, the needles became a tolerable part of dialysis.

When I returned to my home hospital, the technicians and nurses were amazed that I no longer used the numbing medicine, but they weren't surprised that I did it while out of town. Perhaps it was the willingness to take a chance among strangers, one of the technicians commented. If I acted cowardly, screaming and crying, what did it matter? I would have no long-ranged connection with them anyway and therefore wouldn't have to face my cowardice every other day. If things went well, which they did, I could come home with my battle scars like a soldier returning from war with everyone glaring at me in wonder.

That is exactly what happened. When some of the dialysis patients learned that I no longer used lidocaine, they couldn't believe

I could actually endure it. The nurses said it was the best thing to do to preserve my graft, and the tech bowed in acknowledgement of my courage. As I look at my arm now, it has the appearance of someone who has lost her arm in an attack by wild animals and had the limbs reattached, leaving a roadmap of keloids. I wear these scars proudly because they represent a great milestone in my life.

There are also scars on my chest from all the surgeries related to the catheters. When I stand in front of the mirror in the nude, I am a rag doll with needle pricks in my upper chest and my upper and lower left arm. There is beauty here. The keloids on my chest are warrior marks, signaling my battles with renal failure. The browning half moon on my arm is the instrument of war God has given me to stay alive. Sometimes I swing and sway with the melody of my life, putting my arm against my ear and listening to the pulse of my gift. I am alive. There is beauty here. I am a rag doll strengthening myself against the hazards of kidney disease.

Chapter 10

WATER, WATER, EVERYWHERE

With all the information I had collected on renal failure and dialysis, I expected horrendous changes in my life. My days of participating in physical fitness activities would slow and eventually cease. Weight training, step aerobics, running or walking would be just a collage of memories, and I might even become wheelchair bound, as were some of the other patients. I had wondered if I would be able to work—to stand in front of my class with the same dedication and passion, or would I be too exhausted to engage my students?

I had struggled with lethargy, frequent drowsiness, and fatigue for more than a year before I actually went on dialysis. I made excuses for other symptoms of physical deterioration, but I assumed that no matter how poorly I felt before dialysis, it would not compare to the physical decline after dialysis.

I was wrong.

Despite the access difficulties and the dread of going to the facility, after about six weeks of dialysis I became increasingly energetic, alert, and focused. Nearly three months into the treatment, I was able to *do my time* and go directly to the gym, where I worked my way from three days a week on the treadmill to five. Whether or not pre-dialysis physical fitness activities had helped to delay kidney failure longer than the doctors expected, I knew it was certainly one of the keys to easing the potential distress of the dialysis process.

While dialysis enhanced my sense of well-being, it was not an easy life. Not only were the treatments one of two answers to ESRD, with transplants being the other, dialysis demanded rigid discipline and strict adherence to restrictions. Nowhere was this strictness more required than with fluid intake. Physicians and staff constantly encouraged patients to guard against excessive fluid intake, which included liquids and foods with high water content, such as certain fruit and vegetables.

One of the major problems of renal failure is the reduction and eventual cessation of urine and other fluids. During my first year of dialysis, I urinated on my own, but as time passed, the urine output dwindled and finally ceased, thus exacerbating the fluid retention.

Fluid retention is dangerous; excessive retention can be fatal. Patients who gained an inordinate amount of fluid weight talked about their inability to breathe, accompanied by a drowning sensation. Occasionally patients who gained too much fluid were admitted to the hospital as opposed to one of the freestanding dialysis units. The hospital classified those with breathing difficulties as emergency patients because too much fluid had collected around the heart. In such cases, a heart attack and subsequent death are possible.

Physicians are extremely cautious about renal patients and their weight, which is almost always dictated by fluid retention. They determine the patient's dry weight (exact weight without excessive fluid and often calculated with a healthy blood pressure) and encourage them to maintain it. The technicians weigh the patients at each dialysis session, subtract their dry weight from the current weight, and determine how much fluid they will have to remove during the treatment. Patients who maintain a fairly stable weight close to their dry weight face much less danger from the problems associated with fluid retention than those who gain significant weight. Add to this advantage the fact that patients who gain little weight do not have to endure pain from reducing the extra fluid.

Whenever the technicians have to remove excess fluid during the dialysis treatment, the result is agonizing cramping throughout most of the procedure. The pain often begins in the extremities and targets other parts of the body, particularly the calves. Toes involuntary twist and bend, while the hands curl in excruciating knots. The leg muscles tie themselves around ligaments, squeezing and twisting until some patients cry out in agony. More devastatingly, the elimination of excess fluid can reap havoc on the heart muscle, and over time, wear down the organ. Even though some of us could tolerate a greater amount of fluid reduction than others, it is still dangerous to gain too much fluid and horrific when it is removed.

I always tried to remain within the safe limits of fluid intake, but I remember once gaining twelve pounds during a Fourth of July holiday in North Carolina. It was a three-day weekend beginning on Saturday, with daytime temperatures limping between 95-100 degrees and lingering in the low 90's after dark. Still having a modicum of urine output, I forgot about watching my fluid intake and drank whenever I was thirsty.

That Sunday, I attended a wedding in a small country church where the heat had to be at least 10 degrees higher than it was anywhere else. Since there was no air-conditioning, the reception was held under a massive oak tree that shaded us from the sun, but did nothing to protect us from the heat. When the cooks brought out the lemonade with ice bobbing among lemon pulp, and the vapors twirling from plastic cups that had been packed in small freezers, my mouth started to water. As soon as I reached the buffet, I drank, relishing the path forged down my throat and chest and into my stomach by the sweet and cool wetness.

Driving back to Cincinnati, I continued to drink—soda pop, water, iced tea, lemonade, and as much of it as I could, just to fight the long and boring expressway journey. I wasn't thinking.

On Monday when I weighed in, I was astounded at the weight gain—26.4 kilograms or 12 pounds. Having retained this much fluid meant that I must have consumed gallons of liquid, along with the water content of the salads and melons on the menu. The dialysis treatment, however, drained much of the fluid from my system, and in the process, cramped my legs and fingers with such intensity, I could actually see knots in my leg muscles and the bends and twists in my fingers. The on-duty nurse gave me what is known in the dialysis world as a "hot shot"—a saline solution, which minimizes cramping of the muscles. However, by the time the warm liquid crawled through my veins, I was weeping from pain.

From that day on, I learned two important lessons—first, don't drink; sip moderately, and second, pay attention to the advice of the physicians and nurses. The best approach is to measure out the recommended daily fluid allowance and adhere to it. A slight increase or decrease is okay, as long as the fluid is not high in phosphorous or potassium.

The irony is that some fluids, especially water, are good for healthy kidneys, but for diseased kidneys, they can be dangerous. In spite of my tendency towards frequent thirst, I learned to monitor my intake of lemonade, colas (colas should be avoided altogether, given their high phosphorous content), iced tea, water, and even some of the foods with high fluid content such as melons. None of these food products in excess are worth the excruciating and potentially perilous consequences.

In addition to the dangerous results of too much fluid intake, looms the possibility of other equally serious problems. Ingesting too much high potassium foods such as yogurt, tomatoes, oranges and orange juice, raisins, bananas, and other select fruit can damage the heart and in large amounts, stop it. In elevated amounts, foods with high levels of phosphorous—beans, nuts, colas, potatoes, and chocolates for examples, can be equally damaging to certain organs.

After having been on dialysis for a few months, I had learned much about food restrictions, given that the dietician distributed all kinds of literature notifying us of the "acceptable" diet, along with the one that would certainly do us harm. She also checked our blood tests weekly to make sure we were adhering to an acceptable diet. When our various levels were elevated beyond a healthy limit, the dietician would gently chastise us and suggest appropriate food substitutions.

During the nephrologist's weekly visits to the center, the physician checked our blood tests, studied our treatment reports, and reviewed our medications. Of equal importance, he talked to us about our general health and whether or not we were effectively managing dialysis.

Though most of us often thought dialysis was the treatment from hell, we all knew that our healthcare providers were very dedicated to our health and well-being. Undoubtedly, it behooved all of us to pay attention and adhere to the requirements for living well as a dialysis patient.

Chapter 11

AGH! DIALYSIS AND HAIR LOSS, TOO

I'd like to think I approached most of the health scares and anxieties of dialysis with a certain amount of grace. I didn't whine about all the tests, I tried to be stoic in the face of severe pain, and I consented to all the surgeries, even those I questioned. I figured the procedures were simply the aggravating consequences of good dialysis preparation. When I realized the many ramifications of my ESRD, I wanted to travel the road to wellness with dignity. Those who knew of my situation frequently referred to me as a "trooper."

A trooper? Sometimes. There were other times, though, when I sat in the dialysis chair, listening to the discordant sounds of the machine and imagining myself snatching the tubes from my arm and running from the room, screaming like a lunatic. There would be blood draining from the tube, leaving a scarlet trail behind me. I would make it to the door, but as I reached for it, the last bit of energy would fizzle and I would lie in front of the door, bloody and bloated. It was an ugly sight, but I was able at least to visualize turning my back on dialysis, although I knew I never would. I would maintain composure.

But there was one thing I couldn't seem to handle with this imagined self-control. I was losing my hair. In all of my reading about renal failure, dialysis, corresponding medications, diet restrictions, and everything else associated with Chronic Kidney Disease (CKD) and subsequent failure, I had discovered nothing about hair loss.

As I think back on the experience, I laugh at my extreme desperation about hair—the bane of Black women's existence, the albatross around our necks, our "glory" as the old folks used to say. Of all the things I had endured, some gracefully and some childishly, I sank to my lowest level when I started to lose my hair.

I began to notice shedding hair about three months into dialysis. In the mornings especially, I was shocked by strands of hair wrapped in the teeth of the comb and the bristles of the brush. At night, I couldn't believe the curls in the sink and on the pillow. After a while, I began to think I shouldn't comb my hair at all, especially given the way it drifted to my shoulders each time I touched it. Hair seemed to be everywhere excluding my scalp.

When I asked the nurses and doctors if dialysis could cause hair loss, the response was almost always something I already knew—"Maybe, but everybody is different."

"We haven't heard anybody say that," the technicians usually added when I mentioned it to them.

I found that response amazing. Was I the only one on dialysis who was losing hair? My experiences convinced me that there had to be some connection between dialysis and hair loss, since this was the only drastic change to my blood chemistry. Therefore, I took it upon myself to find out if hair loss were a problem unique to me.

When I mentioned hair loss to some of the women patients, they told me they had noticed thinning, but hadn't said anything to the medical staff nor to each other. A couple of them exclaimed that a simple scratch of the head could bring on shedding, and combing was a nightmare. I assumed no one had talked about it because talking made it all too real. Heaven forbid we should be losing hair, along with everything else.

Clearly, there was a connection between dialysis and hair loss, and a few months of dialysis treatments could cause drastic damage to the hair, especially in women.

*****

By December, four months into my dialysis treatments, my hair had thinned to about a third of its pre-dialysis thickness. When I complained over the phone to Jo, my stylist at the time, she said I was probably making more out of the situation than it warranted, and a cut would probably minimize the appearance of "slight" thinning.

However, on the day of my appointment, when she removed my skullcap to take a look, she gasped, "Oh my God! Oh my God!" I could feel the air on my scalp as she exhaled in alarm. Slowly she combed her fingers through my hair and held the loose pieces up to the light. "Oh my God! I had no idea it was this bad!" She shook her head in dismay. "This is bad!"

Her continued exclamations made me feel worse than I did when I entered the shop. Upset, I fought back the tears. "Is it that bad?" I asked meekly, already aware that short of baldness, it couldn't be much worse.

"This is bad! This is really bad!" She explored my hair with her fingers. "I don't think it's a good idea to put any chemical on your hair," she said finally. "It's just not healthy enough."

"Well, you have to do something; I can't do anything with it like this."

She surveyed my hair again, gingerly moving my head from side to side before recommending a conditioner, curl and cut.

When I left the shop, I didn't feel much better than I did when I entered. Jo had pulled some curled hair over the balding spots near the crown, and primped the sides to look as they usually did. This maneuver made only slight improvement. I was losing my hair and the thin spots on the top of my head and the few strands hanging from the back were signs that the worst was yet to come. I was going bald.

With thoughts of baldness uppermost in my mind, I decided I'd get a hair weave. My stylist, who was fast becoming my friend through my hair loss adventure, had just begun weaving after years of working on conventional styles. I didn't know how comfortable she was with the process, but when I questioned her, she reluctantly agreed.

"I don't know if I can do it the way you probably want it," she said.

I insisted. "You can do it." I pointed to my hair. "I can't go around like this."

Thus, a few days after Christmas, when we had extra time away from school, we went in search of hair.

"We'll go look for hair similar in color to your own."

"Yeah," I said. "That's important."

On that Sunday afternoon we planned to buy the hair, there was an ice storm in the city. The streets, covered with about a quarter inch of ice, were slick as onionskin. Driving was ludicrous and walking was just as crazy, but I had to get this hair.

When I stopped by Jo's house on our quest for the hair, her grandson said, "Gramma, where you going in this blizzard?"

"Son, we on a mission!" She wrapped a heavy scarf around her head several times, pulled on her coat and we were out the door.

The two of us drove across town with the desperation of escaped convicts. The car skidded along the streets, but we held on, leaning against the skids and grinding our teeth. Most of the stores had closed because of the weather, but we figured we would take a chance on The Hair Store, a place that focused on hair care products. When we got to the shopping center and parked the car, we tipped, gliding over the ice until we finally slid to the store window.

The store was open, or so we thought. Excitement rose in me like a hot flash. We could see the clerk with her big yellow hair piled on top of her head, straightening hair ornaments and lining wigs along the extended counter. Through the frosty air, we could see our breath as we talked to each other outside the store. The sign said the business didn't close until six. It was now four o'clock. Reaching for the door, I breathed out a mouth of frustration. As I watched the woman moving around in the store, I grabbed the ice-covered knob and turned.

It was locked. We knocked. I started to get nervous. We knocked again.

For a while, the woman with the big hair ignored us. Perhaps she figured nobody in her right mind would have been out in this kind of weather, anyway. We knocked, this time frantically, fiercely, and the woman looked at us and moved slowly to the front, shaking her head no. "We closed at four," she said in a raised voice.

I rubbed the condensation from the glass. Even through the fog from my breath, I could see that the folds around her lips looked like cat whiskers.

"But the sign says six o'clock," Jo argued.

"I know," the woman said. "But since the weather is so bad . . . ice and snow and all, we closed early." She was still shaking her head.

By now, I must have had desperation in my eyes since Jo looked at me, then back at the woman with the big hair. "Ah, have a heart," she pleaded. "We need some hair and we came all the way out here in this weather."

Tears streamed down my cheeks, turning to icicles under my chin. The woman pulled the shade over the door.

"That bitch," Jo snapped through her teeth. "She knows we need that hair and it's only twenty after four." She looked at me with pity in her eyes. "We can always go over to the other market. It's probably open."

"But that store is non-union," I managed to say through a whimper.

"Shit! So what? You better come on here." She hooked her arm in mine and coaxed me away from the door.

We practically slid down the hill to the other store. Here I was going against my political beliefs for some fake hair. I had no shame. I had sunk to an unforgivable level.

Inside, we searched for hair but there was none even close to the color and texture of my own. Flaming red and washed-out yellow weren't going to work for me, so Jo and I decided to wait until the next day to go to some of the stores that specialized in hairpieces, particularly for black women. I left the shopping area with my spirit somewhere among the racks of fake hair.

The next day, we covered almost every black hair care place within a 20-mile radius of my neighborhood. As it had been a great while since I shopped these stores, I was able to observe what I had been reading about in some of the popular magazines. There was not one single store without an Asian standing behind the cash register asking, "May I help you?" Some spoke English better than others, but they were all able to make the point that this was their store, so take it or leave it.

I had some memorable experiences in these stores. Here I am, an African American vigilantly chasing hair to replace that which I had lost through dialysis, and the only African Americans in sight were those shopping in the stores owned by Asians. It didn't matter where I went—to one of the failing neighborhood shopping centers where the only stores remaining were Urban and athletic wear, the Division of Motor Vehicles, and the Five and Dime, or a group of community establishments including a pony keg, bar, church, and a fast food place, there was almost always the Asian hair care shop.

I remember visiting a store reputed to do exceptional business in a shopping center near my neighborhood. Women, old and young, conservative and radical, middle-class and poor, all entered with the intention of combing through jars and cans of chemical hair straighteners, moisturizes and oil treatments, colorful bows and other tacky hair ornaments, earrings and scarfs, wigs and hairpieces.

First, I tried on wigs—the ridiculous and the crude, the long jet-black silky synthetic hair and big bushy brassy naturals. The cashier, sometimes male, sometimes female, always pointed to the hair and said, "This your color. Look good. Good for you, good for you," no matter how stupid it appeared to me. All the time I was trying on the wigs, the proprietor was nearby, watching me with suspicious eyes as I fingered the hair.

Hair—it's been one of the banes of Black women's existence. We dye it, fry it, weave it, curl it, grease it, spray it, twist it, relax it—the list goes on and on, but always we are searching for that perfect look, the one that evokes such admiration as, "Wow! She's got beautiful hair." I was one of these women, wandering through the store rummaging around for this illusion of beauty.

I had also been one of the women lamenting the loss of Black hair care businesses to Asian entrepreneurs. I even refused to go into one of these Asian-run stores, preferring instead to let the stylists and shop owners confront them. However, when I lost my hair to dialysis, I went running to these stores as frantically as one who was on route to collecting a lottery winning. Though I was angry that they stood, crowned in arrogance, watching me as I rambled throughout the store in desperation, I nevertheless patronized them. I thought they had something that could help me.

Standing at the cash register with my pieces of curled hair tucked behind me, I lifted it to the counter while I reached into my purse for my wallet.

"Nice choice," the cashier said, picking it up and searching for the price. "Nice choice. Your color. This your color." In her half-hearted attempt to compliment me, something about her plastic smile said she wanted me to buy this hair and go.

When I left the store with my curled hair tucked neatly in a clear bag, stuck into a paper bag with the company logo on it, I breathed a sigh of relief and hoped I would never have to return.

*****

A few days later, Jo weaved in the store-bought hair. When she finished, I looked like something between an aging rag doll and a cocker spaniel. Though the hair was curly and full, I could see the threading in various places, especially between the bangs and the rest of the hair. I disguised the glaring thread with a bandana whenever I went outside my house.

I was not going to maintain this hairdo because I simply didn't like it. In fact, I hated it. Not only did it look like doll hair, it was itchy and annoying. The style, which reminded me of some of the hairdos of guests on TV talk shows, took on a life of its own. It sat on my head like a bike helmet and looked as if it were ready to take to the air. Then, when my daughter looked at me and burst into laughter, I knew the weave had to go.

In my continuous pursuit of hair, I learned about another hairdresser, one who had amassed an enviable reputation for hair weaving. I arranged to meet with a couple of her clients and observed the "natural look" of her work. In fact, had I not already known the women were wearing weaved hair, I would never have been able to detect it.

I met with the stylist. Upon entering the shop, I could feel an adrenaline rush. There were several stylists around the room working with customers—cutting, weaving, straightening, braiding, perming—doing everything that can be done to black hair. When the woman who turned out to be the one working with me appeared, I felt as if I were waiting to be baptized—to be cleansed and renewed. A small lady with gentle eyes, she seemed to know me before we were introduced. Warmly, she suggested we go to the rear of the salon to talk, a comforting suggestion since I could share more openly in private. In the back of the main room, I pulled off my scarf, revealing my hair. She didn't seem startled, but cuddled my hand in hers.

"Oh yes, dear. We can work with this. We sure can." She spoke calmly as if raising her voice might frighten me.

Gospel music drifted from the front of the salon as my anxiety began to slide from my body like a silk nightgown. It was going to be all right, I told myself. This woman was going to give me some hair and make everything right again.

With the compassion of a chaplain, the stylist told me where to go to get the hair for the weave. She said a dear friend of hers, who owned a shop a few doors from the salon, would be happy to help me select the best hair.

Encouraged that the stylist's friend was the proprietor of the store, I found comfort in knowing I would be able to go into her business and finally get some genuine help from someone who understood African American hair. Relieved that the proprietor of the hair store was, no doubt, African American, I took a deep breath and headed for my dialysis treatment.

A couple of days before the hair appointment, I went to the store the stylist had recommended for the hair. The store—a huge room cluttered with wigs, hairpieces, hair care products, hair ornaments, jewelry, clothes, African woodcarvings, leopard patterned art, had more junk than a county fair. The claustrophobic feel of the place suffocated me and I had the urge to run out to the street. Just as I turned to leave for air, someone said slightly above a whisper, "Need help? Me help you?" I followed the sound to the face of a woman, sixtyish with mixed gray hair with white strands curled around her temples. Her narrow eyes were unfriendly, although her mouth remained a crescent moon the entire time I was in the store. She was Asian.

The woman showed me the hair the stylist had recommended, and tried to encourage me to buy some of her other products. When I declined, she maintained the same smile and bowed her head repeatedly. I left the store resigned to the fact that the day of African American proprietorship of hair care stores had passed, and was now part of the same museums as Black hotels and movie theaters. The reality of this demise smacked me in the face harder than the January wind when I walked out of the store.

Getting a weave turned out to be another of the great learning experiences of my journey. I went into the shop feeling as if I were going to get something that would change my life. Actually, as I reflect on it now, I was so keenly in pursuit of this fake hair that one would have assumed it could restore my kidney function.

As I walked into the shop, I heard the voice of Kirk Franklin's group mingled with the clicking of curling irons and muffled chatter. My stylist beckoned me to the chair as soon as I approached the reception desk in the middle of the waiting room.

"Did you bring the hair?"

"Yes." I handed the bag to her.

She pulled out the mane and turned it over in her hands, examining it. "Yep, this is exactly what I wanted you to get. You're going to be pleased with this."

In a few minutes, she had washed and braided my own hair and prepared it for the weave. She began by attaching the fake hair to the tiny braids around my face, a process requiring her to pull every wild strand of my own hair into the weave. Each time she added hair to the braids, she pulled the hair so tightly my face stretched, and any sagging

I might have had was temporarily swept away somewhere among this heap of hair.

By the time she finished the weave, I had so much hair it weighed down my head. Looking into the stylist's mirror on her dresser, I could barely recognize myself. Not only did I have a pile of medium brown hair glistening against the light in the beauty shop, I also had hair that hung mid-way between my shoulders and my waist. She and I both stared at the hair, her admiring her work, and me wondering who was this woman looking back at me in the mirror.

I left the shop feeling as if I were two feet behind myself, watching this woman in front of me with all this hair. If I tilted my head to either side, the weight of the hair seemed to pull my head in that direction. It felt as if I had a couple of bricks swinging from my scalp. When I met with Jo later in the afternoon, I asked her if she could recognize me anywhere beneath the big mound of hair.

After a few weeks, I was still struggling, trying to get used to the hair. I couldn't pass a mirror without looking at myself, each time hoping to become more accepting of what I saw. Not only did I hate the artificial texture of the hair, I hated its weight, its length, the way its bulk swallowed my face. I even dreamed that a big brown ball of silky hair chased me, then caught and consumed me. When I awakened, hair was spread over the pillow like a fan.

The worst problem with the weave was that it barricaded me from my scalp. Many days I wanted to snatch it from my head and scratch my scalp with the determination and vigor of a dog fighting fleas. When I couldn't do that, I settled for taking a pair of scissors and cutting about six to eight inches of hair, leaving the weave just below my ears and allowing for more access to my scalp.

Increasingly dissatisfied with the weave, I finally saw a television commercial about a hair salon specializing in wigs for those who had suffered hair loss from chemotherapy or some other medical problem. I called the shop, talked to one of the women who worked there, explained my situation and made an appointment. Again, I was on my way to another possible resolution for this hair dilemma, this time with an even greater expectation for a satisfying outcome.

I sat in the waiting room for a short while when the stylist I had talked to on the phone came to greet me. "My name is Sarah," she said, reaching out her hand to me. "Welcome." Her smile appeared genuine.

When I met the stylist, a young white woman, I wasn't sure she had ever worked with African Americans, although she appeared quite confident. After commenting on the exorbitant amount of hair in my present weave, she talked to me about the company's capabilities and decided on the type and color of wig for me.

In less than two weeks, the company had completed the wig. Walking into the front office, I tried to squelch the excitement bubbling in my stomach. Finally I would have the right kind of hair, and it would stand against the ravages of kidney dialysis.

"Come on back." The receptionist smiled warmly. "The wig is here, and I know you're just going to love it."

Trailing the receptionist to the room, I thought about how anxious I was to get a wig—a wig, of all things. Never had I imagined I would even wear a wig, much less feel this kind of anticipation about it.

When the stylist entered with the wig raised before her, I was ecstatic. The deep brown hair was silky and smooth; it glistened against the sunlight that slashed through the window. As I held it in my hands, the hair sliding through my fingers like strands of silk, I had not imagined it so beautiful, and I certainly had not expected I would be as mesmerized by it.

The stylist pushed my chair in front of the big mirror as she prepared to fit the wig snuggly to my scalp. The measurements were accurate and the wig fitted perfectly. There were no revealing signs of artificiality—no divides signaling a simulated part, no gaps around the face, no rows of hair on the scalp, no horsetail stiffness. The wig looked as natural as any wig could, and I left the shop feeling better about my hair than I had since before the initial hair loss. I figured I could live with this look.

I couldn't. Of all the things going on in my life at the time, I had spent days, even weeks, worrying about hair. Such a foolish trivial thing it was, especially given my health dilemmas. The situation wasn't that I hated the wig; I dreaded it, the way I dread weigh-ins in fitness programs. I was also ashamed of it, especially given the priority it had become in my life. How foolish I had been. How much time I had wasted on this quest for hair. Which is why at the end of about six weeks, I came home one afternoon, snatched off the wig and noticed my own hair. It was growing. There were no more bald spots, no areas of fuzzy down, no extreme thinning. I reached to feel the soft dark fleece, letting my fingers roam about my temple, above my ears, around the back of my neck and the top my head. There was hair! I threw up my hands and yelled, "Let there be hair!" In my exuberance, I picked up the wig and took it to the wig stand, where it has been ever since.

I never thought I would be so preoccupied with hair, since I believed I had grown past this kind of worry. With all of my health issues, I had spent too much precious time on what, for me, was a vain pursuit.

Before dialysis, however, my ideals had not been tested. How easy it was to say that I didn't spend an inordinate amount of time fussing with my hair, when I had no problems with it. Then, I could declare that women who are preoccupied with vanity have no sense of self and are searching for meaning in their lives. I had been like the Pharisees, proclaiming, "I thank God I am not like the others." I was proud of my so-called virtues. However, when dialysis caused me to lose my hair, I realized I had as many superficial concerns as anybody else. I, too, had my share of insecurities.

I am now wearing my hair natural. The short kinky black strands curl around the strong subversive gray hair, and I look at it and say, "This is my hair!" Sometimes thinking about how I got to this point, I comb my fingers through it, letting the coarseness scratch the inside of my hands. Dialysis liberated me from an arrogant self-perception, and it also helped me to realize I was subject to some of the same insecurities, uncertainties, and vanities as anyone else. Ironically, it took a major health challenge to help me rethink my priorities.

Angelene J. Hall

Chapter 12

A GLIMPSE OF DIALYSIS CULTURE

In spite of all the turmoil I had experienced as a result of ESRD and subsequent dialysis—surgeries, the physical strain of the procedure, hair loss, frequent swelling of the extremities, occasional nausea and fatigue, and a plethora of other maladies, I finally made an "uneasy" peace with the treatment and settled in at the hospital. The staff moved me into a smaller area away from the extremely ill patients, and I became accustomed to going to the hospital three days a week for "filtering."

After more than a year, I had become familiar with the staff—the technicians, nurses, doctors, social workers, and dieticians. Although we might come into the unit and not see the social worker or the dietician on a given day, we were sure to connect with the technicians and nurses, since they were the ones primarily responsible for our care in the unit.

I had no problems asking the staff questions about the dialysis procedure—what kind of medication the nurses were injecting into the dialysis tubes, its purpose, the dangers of not getting it, the potential side effects, and so on. I was, however, astonished by the number of people who allowed the nurses to inject something into the dialysis tube without ever asking any questions. Rarely did some of them even question their medicinal regimens. In fact, a nurse once told me that many of the patients would rather not know about the medicines; instead, they would prefer the staff took care of the particulars.

Though this *laissez-faire* approach to one's own healthcare is unacceptable to me, I eventually suspected that the unwillingness to take on the work of collecting and understanding information was simply too daunting for some. How many grams of this? How many milligrams of that? When do I take this pill or that pill? What is it for? Is it before a meal or after, and if afterwards, how long? These and similar questions were overwhelming to some patients, and it was apparently easier to leave healthcare matters to the professionals. After all, just showing up three times a week was challenging enough.

Sometimes patients relinquished the control of their care to the doctors and nurses because of their great respect for medical authority. They were awe-inspiring. They could lessen the pain with a pill or reduce the horrendous cramping with a shot into the dialysis tubes. They could do what no one else, other than God, could do. Many of us undergoing dialysis were socialized to believe that doctors were next to God in the healing business. Rarely did we consider what "practicing" medicine really meant, and seldom, if ever, did we think patients were in the position to question their care or challenge medical authority. These professionals were and are the credentialed ones, the ones with the information who are paid to provide healthcare services.

Although professionals provide major services to those seeking health and wholeness, patients have the right and responsibility to be in charge of their own healthcare. If we don't feel comfortable "taking charge," we must certainly participate in the decision-making and resist putting our lives solely in the hands of healthcare providers. We should ask questions when they stick a needle in the dialysis tube to inject iron. Do I need iron? How much and why? This is not to suggest that these providers (doctors, nurses, technicians, etc.) don't have our best interests at heart, but they are people with similar life issues as patients. And, like patients, they have good days and bad days, they forget things, and given the bureaucratic nature of medicine, they rarely have time to get to know each of us as individuals.

Shouldn't a patient know, for example, whether a medication is right for her or him, or one dictated by an insurance company, allegedly to achieve the same effects at half the cost? Isn't it important for dialysis patients to know who makes the decision that technicians inject certain medicines, to the exclusion of others, into the dialysis lines?

Why does the physician choose a specific medication as opposed to another? Does it matter? What are the contraindications for a particular procedure? Is the sonogram or the MRI necessary? Patients need to ask questions, and if they feel inadequate to do so, they should seek someone they trust to speak to the physician.

 As we owe it to ourselves to raise questions about our healthcare, it is critical to remember that few doctors claim to have all the answers. The great divide between the "omniscient" physician and the humbled patient is narrowing, especially with the availability of vast amounts of information. Health magazines, medical websites, and other health media are readily available, even if patients do not care to take advantage of the resources. I am not suggesting we necessarily possess the background to understand the information, but at the very least, the material helps us to formulate questions for our physicians. Even if there ever were a time when physicians' power went unchallenged, it is not the case now with the strangling controls insurance companies exercise over the healthcare industry.

*****

 Assuredly, some of the patients might not have wanted to know the specifics of medication, procedures, and other details of their healthcare, but they were astutely aware of everything else that occurred in the dialysis unit. In fact, dialysis patients at the hospital maintained what I like to call a "dialysis culture." Every morning, the first shift of hospital dialysis patients arrived at the waiting room anywhere from fifteen minutes to a half hour before the technicians opened the door to admit one or two patients at a time. The door is always locked from the inside unless patients are being admitted into the unit. During the time patients waited in the lobby for the technician to call them for treatment, the conversation was like a gathering in a nail salon or barbershop.

 After the acknowledgement of the day's weather, the discussion moved to such topics as, whether or not a dialysis day will fall on a particular holiday, the state of one's graft, which technicians were likely to be working on our shift, the personality of a given technician, and how well she/he could handle the big dialysis needles. The patients often learn something of each other's family, professions, church affiliation, and quite often their politics. Rarely did the conversations turn inwardly, since we ostensibly wanted to keep our deepest selves separate from the hospital.

Another reason many of the patients chose not to become intimately familiar with one another at the hospital dialysis unit is the fear of losing someone to incapacitation or death. It was not uncommon to get used to seeing someone, frequently chatting and developing a certain kind of attachment, only to come into the unit one day and learn that the person has been admitted to the hospital or died.

In a setting such as dialysis, one does not have to be involved in another's life in order to feel a kind of bond; one simply needs the commonality of renal failure. I remember an elderly woman I'll call Mary, who had dialysis the same time I did and usually was sitting in the waiting room when I arrived. Each morning we chatted about nothing particularly important—what we would be doing if we weren't on dialysis, any trips we wanted to schedule, who might be our technician for the day, whether or not the televisions would work adequately, and any other trivia that helped to pass the time. She was always present, until one day she was not. She had suffered a heart attack and died during the night. Her death left a void for all of us in the dialysis room because she was part of the early morning shift. She was one of us.

Most of "us," the first shift patients, and I assume most of the dialysis patients, formed a kind of emotional connection brought on by renal failure and the inconveniences of dialysis. We shared information about the nurses, doctors, technicians, other patients, new research in dialysis and the treatment of kidney diseases. Listening to the conversation, there are certain words that often floated around like the disinfectant smell in the clinic—dry weight, creatinine, BUN, kilos, Calcejex, grafts, catheters, flow (blood flow through the dialysis tubes), fistula, and other terms we learned to associate with renal failure.

Along with the common terms that hovered about the dialysis unit were also the patients' general knowledge of and experiences with the staff. Which doctor is the most competent, most tolerant and patient? Which doctor should we avoid? Which doctor is the best at putting in the graft? Which technician do we want to come for us? We always had an answer to these and similar questions, and perhaps unknowingly, communal talk helped the time pass and made the treatments a little less demanding.

In this setting, information flows, whether factual or part of the folklore. For example, patients are the ones to put the word out on the good nurses as well as the ones who should have gone into a less people-focused profession. A dialysis nurse occupies an extremely important role in the healthcare of dialysis patients. They administer the medication, either in the dialysis tube or in a shot, and they are generally the ones who respond to medical crises, such as fainting spells, chest pains, breathing difficulties, cramping, dangerously low blood pressure-none of which necessarily happen to all patients. The nurses are the ones familiar with patient conditions and usually know how to respond during crises. They make an important difference in the quality of service of dialysis units.

Patients have a major role in helping to shape a nurse's reputation. Quick to pass along information when a nurse is dutiful and tolerant in her handling of patients, they are equally eager to share negative information, such as which nurse can best be described by the "b" word, who is extremely attentive and careful, and who seems to be in another zone while a patient is experiencing some difficulty.

One of the first questions patients raise on their dialysis days is "Who is my nurse today?" Nurses often determine just what kind of dialysis day it is going to be, and it is usually based on something as simple as mood and personality, ability to stick the big needles gently into the graft or fistula, or even their willingness to function effectively with a decrease in staff. Since the nurse is critical to the dialysis patient, any number of nursing issues can trigger either a good dialysis day or the dialysis day from hell.

As with the nurses, the technicians do not escape the severity of patient scrutiny. Actually, technicians often reap more wrath or praise than either the doctors or nurses. Usually the technicians get the machines ready for dialysis, bring the patients into the unit, take their weight, blood pressure, temperature, check their lungs and heart, and hook them to the machines. Before hooking the patients to the machines, however, the technicians locate their dialysis access and then stick the needles into the site. Unless the patient has a catheter or insists on lidocaine, the technicians must use the 15-gauge needle if the access is healthy. If not, the nurse or technician adjusts the needle accordingly.

It is quite easy for technicians to get a draconian reputation, which means they are horrendous with the needles, or as the saying goes in the dialysis culture, "they have blood on their hands." There is an art to inserting the needles with the least amount of pain and not all of the technicians or the nurses have mastered that art. Some of them use the needle the same way they would use an ice pick. In fact, some patients request not to be stuck by certain technicians, while others endure the pain and subsequently spread disparaging information about the technician. If technicians talk too much or too little, treat patients with disrespect or patronizing admiration, speak to them as if they are children or deaf or both, or forget that dialysis patients are human beings struggling with very real challenges, they are headed for the gossip slush pile.

Since dialysis technicians interact with the patients more than anyone else, receiving more of the criticism, favorable or unfavorable, is a natural progression. It appeared that the market for technicians was booming when I was a patient. With the high turnover rate among the technicians, management hired new technicians regularly. A new employee is a good thing, though, especially since the ratio of patients to technicians often rose as high as 5 to 1.

However, it didn't appear as if new technicians received the kind of intensive training necessitated by the complexity of the dialysis process. Eight weeks of on-the-job training, a training manual, a series of tests, and participation in a two-week in-class training, are not exactly what I consider extensive training. Yet, these healthcare providers expected the technicians to master a very intricate and detailed process in two or three months. Sometimes tutored by a nurse, but more often by a seasoned technician, the new hire essentially learned by doing and reading a training manual. I was often amazed at the progress of some of the new hires, although there were a few who realized working in dialysis was not for them and quit before the end of the probation period.

No dialysis patient wants to see a new tech approaching her/his station with eyes hooded in uncertainty and intimidation. Initially fearful of hurting the patients with such gigantic needles, the new technicians are often uncomfortable sticking the patients, even if she or he has worked in dialysis for a few months. Some of us have talked about the need for a detailed orientation on dialysis and patient care, including sensitivity training, several months of intensive training in the dialysis process, and certainly some coaching in general patient care.

I've often wondered if dialysis management ever considered having potential employees engage in some form of psychological testing to determine their temperament, endurance, patience, communication skills, and sensitivity to the human condition. In other words, shouldn't there be something built into the renal care system which allows potential employees the chance to determine if they are suited to be dialysis technicians? Such a procedure might alleviate the high turnover rate among dialysis technicians.

*****

People who work in dialysis, especially the technicians with minimal healthcare training, need not only a comprehension of the science of dialysis, but also some understanding of people coping with a chronic illness. Unless and until a dialysis patient receives a kidney transplant, she/he is dependent on a machine three days a week at least three to four hours or longer at each setting. Sometimes the realization of this dependency affects the patients psychologically, causing them to shift emotionally from sadness to anger to resentment, and technicians should be able to respond to these changing moods. Technicians who respond to dialysis patients as if they are merely chair #2 or chair number #3 might as well be working in an automobile manufacturing plant, where cars are assembled and prepared for the market. Snatching someone from the streets, as it were, who simply needs a job is not the way to recruit dialysis personnel.

Complaints about such matters are a natural part of the dialysis culture. We talk. We listen. We watch. Although most of us generally hate the three-day trek to the dialysis units, we nevertheless understand that our life depends on the artificial kidney.

We want all those who work with, around, and for us to realize their role in saving our lives. We grumble when technicians and nurses are late for work and therefore don't get the machines set up for us to begin dialyzing on schedule. Starting late means finishing late. The night shift's negligence in getting the machines set up should not be our problem. We don't need to hear the technicians complain about what last night's shift didn't do, or how sleepy they are at such an early morning hour. We have a much bigger problem—renal failure, which should take priority, especially in the dialysis culture.

I am a part of this culture. I am a dialysis patient and I have finally accepted my renal failure. I do not see myself as ill because I am not ill. Rather, I have a physical challenge for which there is treatment. I have felt much better since I began dialysis and have long since resumed my normal activities—aerobic exercise, weight training, swim classes, and sometimes even running. In fact, occasionally after my dialysis treatment and my standing systolic is less than 100 (the minimum number of the systolic pressure before one can leave the dialysis unit), I perform between 15-20 jumping jacks to elevate the pressure. With injections from an attached bag of saline attached, I usually get the pressure elevated in less than two minutes.

Of course, many nights I asked God to let me wake up the next day with fully functioning kidneys, but God obviously wanted me to see the miracle He had already provided—dialysis. I thanked Him for it.

*****

I spent a year and a half on dialysis at the hospital, during which time I came to know what to expect, whom to embrace, whom to shun. I finally came to understand that I still have a very precious life, and that God has given me the strength and courage to move on, despite my reliance on the machine. I came to recognize my connection to other patients at the dialysis unit in the hospital, and I realized I had developed a special fondness for some of the nurses and technicians. The social workers and dieticians were also helpful and responded promptly to any needs I had.

Not only did I make peace with dialysis, I began to understand that dialysis was not some kind of punishment exercised by God against me. I experienced renal failure, but only after I had been diagnosed with chronic kidney disease over a quarter of a century ago. This situation could have been much worse. Unlike some dialysis patients, dialysis didn't make me sick, and for that I am especially grateful. God was with me as I dealt with dialysis, and I knew that unless and until I received a kidney transplant, dialysis would be just another part of my life.

Chapter 13

THE KIDNEY FACTORY: DIALYSIS FOR PROFIT AND THE OUTPATIENT CLINICS

Making peace with dialysis didn't end my tests of endurance. One Wednesday morning, after the techs had connected the tubes to my arm and I had settled into my dialysis chair, I thought I would read before sleep came. I usually pulled the small television in front of me to catch the day's weather predictions and early news, which frequently made me drowsy. This time, however, I ignored the television in favor of working on a manuscript I had been editing.

While I flipped through a couple of pages searching for the area I had marked, "Start here," the social worker entered the pod.

"You are going to be mad with me," she said, resting a hand on each hip. "When I tell you what I got to tell you, you're not going to like it."

I couldn't imagine what she could have been referring to. I hadn't asked for any travel arrangements, so she couldn't be talking about botched travel schedules or a lack of vacancies at a given cite. "What's wrong?"

"You are leaving the hospital," she blurted. "Being transferred to the out-patient facility." She spoke fast, as if she needed to get all of this out before I could respond.

I tried to say something, but the words wouldn't come. My mouth dried and my tongue seemed paralyzed. I was devastated. This was the last thing I expected or wanted.

"It's Tuesday, Thursday and Saturday, instead of Monday, Wednesday and Friday, but at least you got a 5:00-8:00 AM time slot. You like early," she reminded me.

DUCK SUMMER: *MY ODYSSEY AS A DIALYSIS PATIENT*

No matter how hard I tried to hold them back, tears slid down my cheeks. "But I don't want to leave," I finally mumbled. "I want to stay here."

The social worker shook her head in empathy. "I'm so sorry," she said. "I tried to convince them to keep you here, but the doctor said you had to go . . . said you should have been gone months ago because you don't need the hospital."

I could feel her eyes on me.

"At least that's a good thing, right? You are well enough to be transferred to one of the outpatient sites, and you have been in good shape for a long time now."

Even in my tears, I could feel her waiting for me to say something.

"Tell you the truth," she continues. "I don't know how you managed to stay here this long." She still waited, but I could tell her patience was waning as her tone became a little edgy. "You might as well get ready."

I finally bowed my head in agreement, but I was still crying.

Throughout the rest of my time at the unit that morning, nurses and technicians stopped to say goodbye and that they would miss me. They reminded me that going to one of the clinics meant I was a healthy dialysis patient and my leaving would provide space for a patient who needed the specialized services. I had stayed at the hospital longer than most of the healthy patients, anyway, possibly because whenever the subject of transfers came up, the staff, for whatever reason, had not pointed to me. But the time had finally caught up with me and I had to go.

My attitude was no different from some of the other patients, who also didn't want to leave the hospital. The hospital is where many of us receive our dialysis initiation. It is often where we adjust to the procedure and where we are treated with special attention. There, we get to know the healthcare providers in dialysis, and what to expect. We establish our treatment routines, perhaps begin to feel at least a measure of acceptance with the process, and acquire a special kind of relationship with the healthcare providers, particularly those who go out of their way to be kind. Finally, there were things about the hospital that gave some of us the notion that dialysis was not necessarily permanent, perhaps the myth that hospitalization meant recovery.

Having slowly adjusted to the special care provided by hospital dialysis, which catered to the ill and disabled patients, most of us rejected the idea of leaving for some unknown dialysis clinic. We had dodged some of the horror we had learned about these centers through the "renal grapevine," random publications, and even our own minimal experiences.

It was now time for me to say good-bye to the staff and patients to whom I had become accustomed. I was waving farewell to the safety and comfort of the familiar—the heated blankets, the small cups of soft drink, the weekly Monday morning visit from a retired nephrologist still working with renal patients, a wheelchair patient who made us all laugh, etc. I was leaving everything I had finally accepted as part of my changed world.

Perhaps my sense of dread in leaving the hospital also came from the perception of freestanding dialysis centers I developed during my travels. I started to believe the centers were in the business of dialysis. I appreciated that such facilities did, in fact, exist because hospitals were not prepared to care for the exorbitant number of patients with renal failure. Though dialysis clinics were a lifeline to millions of people, I still didn't want to be one of the patients.

Clinics seemed to increase my anxiety about dialysis because they reminded me that I was on a path that might never end. Each day,

DUCK SUMMER: *MY ODYSSEY AS A DIALYSIS PATIENT*

I watched patients, many of whom were African American, sit around the room in chair after chair, sleeping, watching television, cramping, and even moaning against the beeping, buzzing and clanging of the machines. Rarely was there a vacant chair, and even when a patient skipped a treatment, the staff called in another patient from a later shift to take the dialysis chair. Initially, the dialysis unit reminded me of an assembly line with the sights, sounds, and feel of automation.

One morning as I dressed for dialysis, my husband teased, "Don't tarry, you gotta hurry to the kidney factory." Constantly encouraging me to look at dialysis as another one of the challenges of life that I could handle, he frequently tried humor to cheer me. For example, his way of encouraging me was to look at my determination to follow my renal diet as "hitting it out of the park." When I starting on another activity after returning home from dialysis, he told me I had certainly hit a home run that particular day. Though I occasionally tired of his baseball metaphors, the image of the dialysis facility as a kidney factory was intriguing and I asked for an explanation.

He reminded me of a time when we were in Georgia and he had accompanied me into the dialysis center. In the treatment room, he noticed how the machines were lined up around the room with beepers and buzzers alternatively making discordant sounds. The arrangement of the machines, along with people moving about like wound up pieces of equipment, presented the image of a factory right out of a Dickens' novel.

I had heard about the outpatient centers since my first few weeks on dialysis. According to folklore, streaked with a modicum of truth, some of the units really did run like factories. Patients came into the dialysis area, were hooked to the machines, dialyzed their required time, and left the unit, unless their blood pressures were too low. When the next patients were scheduled, they repeated the process, and the routine continued until late into the evening when the facility closed. Patients experiencing difficulties in breathing, blood pressure, fainting, nausea, or other health issues had to remain until their complications subsided.

I am not suggesting that the units don't seem to care about the health of the patient. Most of them do the best they can, given the seemingly inadequate number of staff for the vast number of patients. Also, the transient nature of technicians, along with their questionable training, poses a threat to the healthcare provided by the freestanding units.

These freestanding units are, by and large, for-profit centers. As such, the staff had to account for everything from Band-Aids to facial tissue. Rarely did I frequent a unit with adequate staff, and often the workers were stretched thin enough to snap. Unlike the hospitals, there were no cotton sheets to cover the plastic recliners, no warm blankets to protect patients from the massive drop in body temperature during treatment, and no pillows to aid in neck and shoulder comfort unless patients brought them from home. For cover, the units provided paper-thin sheets of blue plastic, and there was no such thing as a "free drink" in the outpatient units. So when the technicians completed readying the machines and asked, "What else can I get for you?" the patients responded, "Nothing, thank you," because there *was* nothing. Some of us brought our own blankets and pillows, our own drink, and even our own facial tissue unless we wanted to use the Center's, which was almost as rough as newspaper.

I had been at a Center since the end of March 2000. It took only about eight to ten minutes to get there and I usually left home around 4:45 in the morning. Although the nurses and technicians were generally competent, it took months to adjust to not being at the hospital. The 16-3 ratio of patients to staff represented the never-ending problem of too few staff and too many patients.

Since dialysis chairs were stationed around and against the wall facing the center of the fairly large room, some patients found it difficult to establish any connection with others. Many patients beginning dialysis on the 5 and 5:15 A M shifts usually fell asleep within ten to fifteen minutes after their arrival. Rarely was there much time to socialize in the waiting room because patients were usually there fifteen to twenty minutes before their scheduled hook-up time. Things were often rushed, especially if any staff or patients were late because the technicians were trying to get the people hooked to the machine in the allotted time period. The unit appeared safe and dialysis was generally efficient, but sometimes the environment appeared cold and detached.

I had been used to sleeping much of the time at the hospital, but when I was assigned to the Center, I was awake during most of the treatment. It took a couple of months before I began to get adjusted to the new setting, and even another month or more before I was able to shed the feeling of being a stranger in an alien land. However, I frequently reminded myself that dialysis was not a social affair in some posh hotel where we went to relax three times a week. This was a hemodialysis unit and I was a patient.

*****

"I-am-a-dialysis-patient," I frequently repeated to myself, especially after I began to dialyze at the Center. However, few people actually seemed to know what that meant. I remember being introduced to a friend of one of my colleagues, during which time the subject of my dialysis came up. The woman to whom I was introduced cried out, "You're on dialysis? My God, why?" Her exclamation, along with her befuddled expression, seemed to suggest that either my doctors and/or I had arbitrarily selected dialysis as a way of life. Apparently, the woman knew little or nothing about dialysis, other than it must be a horrible ordeal.

These and similar responses to my life as a hemodialysis patient, made me more aware of the loneliness, which was often compounded by a sense of otherness. Among people who were generally unfamiliar with dialysis, I felt I was the outsider, the woman who had to bond with a machine three days a week in order to stay alive. I was the one who had this special "condition."

During the initial stage of dialysis, most of my friends and acquaintances, those even vaguely aware of dialysis, looked upon my having to undergo the therapy as a horrible experience that would render me weak and sickly, unable to function without assistance, and certainly incapable of maintaining a job.

However, my friends were taken aback to see that I didn't appear frail, lethargic or otherwise physically challenged; I was instead, energetic and enthusiastic about life. In fact, after a couple of months of treatment in the hospital, I had more energy than I had experienced in a very long time. Some of my colleagues seemed amazed that I had not been in and out of the hospital (at least that's what they thought) or that I was able to maintain my normal activities. Not many people knew about the very early days of dialysis, with all the hospitalizations, surgeries and other health challenges, but they knew I had been ill and assumed this procedure must have cured the ailment.

Others have looked at dialysis as a cure to kidney disease rather than a long-term treatment. Dialysis does not cure end-stage renal disease; instead, it replaces the function of the kidney until the patient undergoes a kidney transplant. In those cases where a transplant is not recommended, the patient is dialyzed for life.

After I went into end-stage renal failure, I gave considerable thought to how I truly felt about dialysis. After almost three years of treatment, I realized I had a love-hate relationship with it. Blessed to live during a time when medicine is advanced to the stage where people can thrive and live productive lives in spite of renal failure, I had heard about the times when the mortality rate for dialysis patients was very high. Less than forty years ago, for example, dialysis carried greater risks and unpredictability, leaving patients to rely on half-day therapies with far greater complications than we currently face. Today, dialysis is less demanding on the body and allows many patients to live a relatively normal life.

However, as I praise dialysis everyday for its life-sustaining benefits, I have often looked at it with a sense of fear and dread. Thinking of myself as dependent on this therapy, I have thought of it as a kind of prison sentence, a punishment for something of which I am completely unaware. On some mornings when I sat in the lobby waiting for one of the technicians or nurses to come for me, I fantasized about the days before dialysis and asked myself, what did I do with the three and a half hours I currently spend in the dialysis chair? I must certainly have been doing something wonderful, if nothing more than sleeping. I dreamed of the days when a diet cola was as common a couple of times a day as brushing my teeth, and taking a vacation was a simple process if I had the time and money. Now, taking a vacation longer than two days required my speaking to the social worker about scheduling the procedure at the destination or one as close by as possible, assuming the centers had a vacancy. Although the dialysis staff can usually arrange for travel, if given at least two to three weeks notice, I think that deep down, I very much resented the inconvenience.

Another concern about dialysis is the primitive nature of the process. I mentioned before the advancement in dialysis over the last few decades, but given the progress of medical procedures in general, dialysis is still a very primitive process. Considering the various computer-generated and computer-enhanced procedures, it seemed extremely backwards that patients with grafts and fistulas are stuck with needles the size of a small Phillips screwdriver twice for each setting three times a week. If a computer can keep a jet in the air or a train on the tracks or information in the clouds, why can't the same technology be used to develop a more user-friendly method of performing kidney functions?

During some of my more cynical moments, I have suspected

that somewhere in a remote laboratory at some university science/medical lab is a computer-generated kidney small enough to fit inside the body and replace the current dialysis system. Scientists are not allowed to present this technology to the public because such a discovery would render the institution of dialysis, which includes pharmaceutical companies, dialysis machine and artificial kidney manufacturers, for-profit dialysis centers, stocks and all other profits from end stage renal disease, about as valuable as junk bonds.

Dialysis is an expensive treatment with a month's therapy for the individual patient ranging from $10,000 to $12,000, a fee which might not include weekly blood tests, doctors' review of blood tests, bi-monthly visits of doctors' assistants to the dialysis center, and any of the many tools of the process. It should be noted, however, than Medicare and individual health insurance assume a significant part of the costs for the treatments. During my tenure, for example, my employment insurance was key to my ability to pay for the treatments. For the first 30 months, my insurance was the primary payer, after which Medicare became primary. For those who are uninsured, Medicare Part B is critical to their treatments. Costs fluctuate with the changing healthcare climate as indicated in various consumer publications. The "miracle chip," as I like to call it, would dismantle would be a miracle for the dialysis patient and probably help to dismantle what I suspect is a profitable system.

The idea of dialysis for profit leaves me feeling as if somebody out there is making money from the illness of millions of people throughout the country. I am aware that looking at dialysis from the dialysis chair lends itself to oversimplification, which is probably the best justification for a more thorough orientation at the onset of the experience. Granted, all that I probably do not know about dialysis as a system of healthcare could fill a library, but my perspective is that of the patient, which means I view everything about dialysis from the dialysis chair. Given that patients do not get any information that healthcare providers see as irrelevant to our diagnosis, it is not surprising that cynicism can attack our thinking as fiercely as disease attacked our kidneys.

I can recall the number of times the word, "business," has entered my discussion of medicine. Conversations about health insurance companies inevitably lead to dialogue about the business of medicine and how hospitals, in spite of their technological advancements and abilities to save lives, seem to be sinking in bureaucratic quicksand. However, for me, these were general conversations, and although engaging, meant little more than the ranting of people dissatisfied with the administration of healthcare.

As an end stage renal disease patient, I have begun to take the word, "business," more seriously. With the draconian costs of healthcare and providers having to account for everything from Band-Aids to the plastic sheets that cover the dialysis chairs, dialysis centers are forced to squeeze the green from the dollar. I worry, for example, that in most outpatient dialysis centers, the administrative demand to keep every dialysis chair filled will drain the integrity from the process.

If a center has fifteen to twenty chairs, each occupied, then there should be adequate staff to accommodate the patients, therefore enhancing the quality of care and the availability of options for them. If one patient is distressed with severe cramping while another is losing consciousness, then each needs a technician or nurse. Patients should not have to stand in line to acquire the necessary attention.

However, if the motivation is profit, patients will suffer the risks of cost-cutting healthcare practices. Dialysis units are healthcare facilities—life-supporting facilities. They are not Dickensian warehouses with assembly lines and piece workers. If the interests of the patients are at the center of the system, then everything about dialysis will be developed with patients in mind, which of course, speaks against dialysis for profit.

Angelene J. Hall

Chapter 14

KIDNEY TRANSPLANTS

Writing this memoir on my ESRD and subsequent hemodialysis has given me an invaluable opportunity to reflect on living with a chronic illness. When a kidney is barely working, perhaps at a five percent level, worse or not at all, many other things can go wrong with the body. Kidneys affect blood pressure, bone density, vascular health, heart condition and a number of other bodily functions. In brief, kidneys are major organs, which if damaged by high blood pressure, diabetes, other illnesses, or just bad luck, can result in a drastic life change.

As noted in this discussion, ESRD patients can opt to do nothing, in which case death is imminent, or they can choose one of the forms of dialysis—hemodialysis, peritoneal, or overnight home dialysis. Any form of dialysis is very expensive. According to some reports, dialysis can cost upwards of "$77,000 a year per patient, or more than $20 million per year."[3] Medicare helps significantly with the costs for those without insurance, and after the first thirty months of treatment, assumes a large percent of the cost for those with insurance. For example, as a faculty member, I had very good insurance through the University, which picked up most of the expenses for dialysis for the first thirty months, after which Medicare became the primary carrier.

Despite the financial assistance available for dialysis, the best possible choice for an ESRD patient is transplantation. A successful transplant promises a restoration of health, along with freedom from all dialysis tests and surgeries. The transplant recipient can, ideally, say goodbye to clinics, machines, needles, meds, de-clotting centers, rigid food restrictions, wretched fluid limitations and guarded time management. Of particular importance, transplants can significantly curtail the

---

3   Consumer Reports on Health, "Caring for Your Kidneys," Vol. 23, Number 8, August 2011.

physical strains on the body as a consequence of dialysis. This miraculous gift promises health and hope—a new life, and above all, a kind of freedom that only dialysis patients can appreciate.

I am pleased to know that there is significant research occurring in the area of stem cell reproduction. One day, there might be the miracle of cell regeneration for patients with ESRD. It is also likely that dialysis, as we know it, might develop into an even more advanced and less invasive and repetitive procedure. I get excited when I hear even the spotty news about the possibility that one day healthy organs developed in laboratories might replace diseased ones. As current scientific and anecdotal information indicate, dialysis is light years more advanced and progressive than it was in its earlier days. Given existing research and testing in nephrology, it is therefore reasonable to assume that we can soon expect miracles in this area.

Today, however, our miracle is organ transplantation.

*****

As a dialysis patient, I learned much about the healthcare system, particularly that part of it relative to kidney transplants. Medical pamphlets, articles on transplantation for the general public, newsletters and other literature from the Kidney Foundation, and conversations with physicians and nurses, are readily available to patients seeking information on transplants. Such information is especially important to anyone thinking about a transplant because it outlines the process the patient has to follow. From being listed, to actually going through the post-transplant process, the details of transplantation are readily available.

In order for ESRD patients to have greater access to healthy kidneys, there needs to be three things—good overall health of the patient, availability of healthy kidneys, and patience. It takes patience to go through the process of getting listed for a transplant, which occurs only after a series of tests to determine the patient's eligibility.

There are also at least three interviews, one with the transplant surgeon and the others with kidney doctors and staff. Then, if all goes well, the patient is placed on the transplant list.

I lost two opportunities for placement on the transplant list. The thyroid problem, which developed the same year I began dialysis, precluded consideration for a transplant for a couple of years. After having been listed for about a year, I developed breast cancer, which was diagnosed as pre-stage one and early enough that the medical profession could not determine whether or not it was hormone specific. This early diagnosis was extremely advantageous to my general health, but it kicked me off the list again for another two years.

I am now waiting for a kidney transplant. I have gone through the testing and have been listed again. Having completed the transplant interviews, I understand that the transplant is not a cure-all, but it will provide the kind of freedom that is not allowed by dialysis. As I wait for a kidney, I'm anxious, and I'm sometimes discouraged, wondering if it will ever happen.

Although I can't always keep my spirits as elevated as I would like, I try to look at my life as one filled with opportunities and possibilities. I am, after all, alive. I have a life, in spite of dialysis. Each day is a new beginning, another chance to make the most of being alive. With family, work, church, my writing, fitness routines, one season's going into another, and all the other blessings, I strive to be the best I can and contribute the most I can. Renal failure has not stolen my life. Rather, it has shown me that physical challenges don't always mean physical, emotional and psychological immobilization.

My appreciation and love for life during this journey cannot be attributed solely to my own fortitude. Renal failure and subsequent dialysis have added significantly to my growing relationship with God. He has taught me how to approach this journey, to understand that in spite of its ease or difficulty, He is there, pointing me in the right directions and often carrying me through the foggiest of times. Recognizing how God has been with me through my triumphs and struggles—shouldering me, laughing with me, and sometimes letting me find the way He has established for me, I know what an integral part of my life He is.

In many ways, through information, doctors, technologies, hospitals, patients, dialysis, family, friends and other support systems, God has always been with me.

Angelene J. Hall

Epilogue

I came home Monday morning, September 13, 2004, after my three hour and a half treatment and went immediately to my elliptical machine. After a half hour, I sat at my desk wiping perspiration from my face and staring at the keyboard. The phone rang.

"Hello?"

"This is Kidney and Hypertension. Is Angelene available?"

"This is she."

"I'm calling because I think we have a kidney for you."

For a minute, I was afraid to speak. This was a dream and if I said something, it would fade, and I would be left with only a memory and the disappointment of thinking I had gotten a kidney when I really didn't. I couldn't bear that.

"Are you there?"

"Yes, yes, I'm here." My pulse raced. "Is this really true?" I asked before thinking. "I've waited so long."

"Well, we think so. But remember, you had some problems that kept you off the list for a while. Did you eat anything?'

My throat immediately dried and I tried to swallow. "No, no, I didn't."

"Good. We want to give the kidney to you or to this other person, but we think he might have a problem."

"When will I know for sure?" I took a deep breath, trying to settle down.

"I'm going to check and call you right back to let you know for sure."

DUCK SUMMER: *MY ODYSSEY AS A DIALYSIS PATIENT*

"I'll be right ---." The dial tone cut off my comment. I wanted to tell him, "I'll be right here beside the phone. Waiting."

I was afraid to move and I prayed no one would call me to tie up the phone, not even long enough for me to say I was waiting for a call.

After about twenty minutes, the phone rang again. My hands began to sweat. My right hand stiffened and it seemed I couldn't move it. Somehow, though, before I realized it, I heard the doctor's voice.

"It's yours . . . the kidney is yours. So get to the hospital."

"Thank you! Thank you! Thank you so much!" I put the phone on the receiver, slowly, as if to move rapidly would awaken me and I would find that all this was a dream. I put my hand on my chest, feeling for my heartbeat. It all seemed so unreal. So scary, so exciting, so joyful.

I called my husband, told him the news and heard myself yell, as if I wanted to make sure he heard me. "I'll just drive myself to the hospital. I'll have the car and I can drive myself home when it's over." I didn't realize that a transplant was as intensive a procedure as it was. In the excitement, I guess I assumed it was a same day procedure and would take a short time. Crazy!

"I know you're excited, but you gotta calm down," he said, speaking with all deliberateness. "Drive yourself and I'll get someone to bring the car home."

"I can't believe this is really happening! Is it really happening after all this time?" I could feel myself jumping up and down, the perspiration from the excitement and the elliptical machine draining from my scalp and down my face.

"Calm down, now. Yes, this is real. Very real."

Angelene J. Hall

The Author

    Angelene J. Hall was twelve years old when her parents left sharecropping for a small town in the Piedmont region of North Carolina. From a sharecropper's daughter to Professor Emerita, University of Cincinnati, she taught courses in black creative expression, including especially African American literature, and wrote and presented both fiction and scholarship. During her tenure at the University, she went into renal failure and ultimately spent six years (1998-2004) on kidney dialysis. DUCK SUMMER, her most recent work, represents her efforts to use her experiences with ESRD to educate the public about renal decline and ultimate failure, dialysis, and the urgency of organ donation.

www.angelenejhall.com

Made in the USA
Charleston, SC
28 November 2015